thefacts

Polycystic ovary syndrome

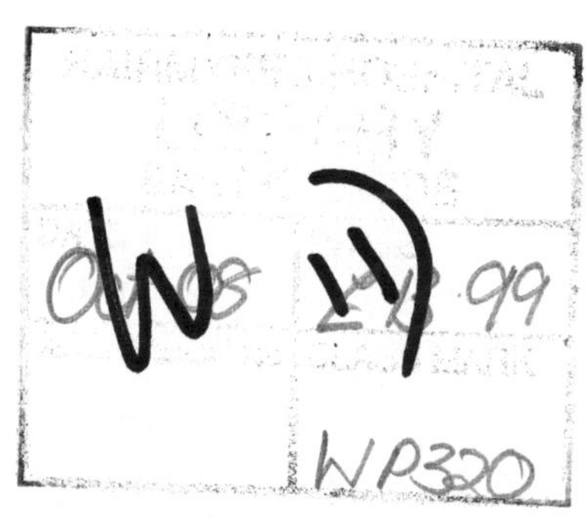

Published and forthcoming titles in **the facts** series

Eating disorders: the**facts**
FIFTH EDITION
Abraham and Llewelyn-Jones

Sexually transmitted infections: the**facts**
SECOND EDITION
Barlow

Autism and Asperger syndrome: the**facts**
Baron-Cohen

Back and neck pain: the**facts**
THIRD EDITION
Jayson

Kidney failure: the**facts**
Cameron

Chronic fatigue syndrome: the**facts**
Campling

Living with a long-term illness: the**facts**
Campling

Prenatal tests: the**facts**
De Crespigny

Obsessive-compulsive disorder: the**facts**
THIRD EDITION
de Silva and Rachman

Muscular dystrophy: the**facts**
THIRD EDITION
Emery

Alcoholism: the**facts**
THIRD EDITION
Goodwin

The pill and other forms of hormonal contraception: the**facts**
SIXTH EDITION
Guillebaud

Myotonic dystrophy: the**facts**
Harper

Epilepsy: the**facts**
SECOND EDITION
Hopkins

Ankylosing spondylitis: the**facts**
Khan

Prostate cancer: the**facts**
Mason

Multiple sclerosis: the**facts**
FOURTH EDITION
Matthews

Essential tremor: the**facts**
Plumb

Huntington's disease: the**facts**
Quarrell

Panic disorder: the**facts**
SECOND EDITION
Rachman

Tourette syndrome: the**facts**
Robertson

ADHD: the**facts**
Selikowitz

Down syndrome: the**facts**
SECOND EDITION
Selikowitz

Dyslexia and other learning difficulties: the**facts**
SECOND EDITION
Selikowitz

Schizophrenia: the**facts**
SECOND EDITION
Tsuang

Depression: the**facts**
Wassermann

Motor neuron disease: the**facts**
Talbot and Marsden

Borderline personality disorder: the**facts**
Krawitz and Jackson

Thyroid disease: the**facts**
FOURTH EDITION
Vanderpump and Tunbridge

Polycystic ovary syndrome: the**facts**
Elsheikh and Murphy

thefacts

Polycystic ovary syndrome

DR MOHGAH ELSHEIKH

Centre for Endocrinology and Diabetes,
Royal Berkshire Hospital, Reading, UK

MISS CAROLINE MURPHY

Centre for Endocrinology and Diabetes,
Royal Berkshire Hospital, Reading, UK

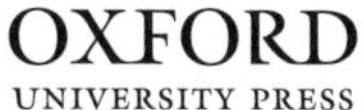

OXFORD
UNIVERSITY PRESS

Great Clarendon Street, Oxford OX2 6DP

Oxford University Press is a department of the University of Oxford.
It furthers the University's objective of excellence in research, scholarship,
and education by publishing worldwide in

Oxford New York

Auckland Cape Town Dar es Salaam Hong Kong Karachi
Kuala Lumpur Madrid Melbourne Mexico City Nairobi
New Delhi Shanghai Taipei Toronto

With offices in

Argentina Austria Brazil Chile Czech Republic France Greece
Guatemala Hungary Italy Japan South Korea Poland Portugal
Singapore Switzerland Thailand Turkey Ukraine Vietnam

Oxford is a registered trade mark of Oxford University Press
in the UK and in certain other countries

Published in the United States
by Oxford University Press Inc., New York

British Library Cataloguing in Publication Data

Data available

Library of Congress Cataloging in Publication Data

Data available

Typeset by Newgen Imaging Systems (P) Ltd., Chennai, India
Printed in China
on acid-free paper by
Phoenix Offset

ISBN 978–0–19–921368–9 (Pbk.: alk paper)

10 9 8 7 6 5 4 3 2 1

Contents

Part 3
Weight management in polycystic ovary syndrome

Part 1

About polycystic ovary syndrome

Introduction

Polycystic ovary syndrome (PCOS) is the most common hormonal disorder to affect women. It can reduce fertility and it can affect appearance by causing acne, excess facial and body hair growth, or scalp hair thinning. Consequently the symptoms associated with PCOS can affect self-esteem, and some women may even suffer from depression because of the severity of these symptoms. This book aims to help you understand PCOS, gives you practical advice on how to control the symptoms, and aims to help you lead a more satisfying life. The book also provides an in-depth guide to all available medical and natural treatments so that you are well informed when you go to your doctor or therapist. Many of you with PCOS have problems with weight gain and difficulty losing weight. Symptoms also tend to be more severe if you are overweight. Furthermore, PCOS can increase your risk of developing diabetes and possibly heart disease, particularly if you are overweight or obese. Research has shown that through weight loss and maintaining a healthy lifestyle, your symptoms can be improved and your health risks minimized. This book therefore has a large section dedicated to weight management, primarily by incorporating the low glycaemic index (GI) principles to diet. The treatment chapters also contain personal success stories from women who were treated at the PCOS clinic in Berkshire using the methods recommended by the book. The final section in the book aims to be a reference source for women with PCOS and includes GI and calorie tables, and a list of useful websites. We hope that this book will be an invaluable resource for you, will empower you with the knowledge to take control of your health, and will provide you with strategies to cope with the effects of living with PCOS.

1

What is polycystic ovary syndrome?

Key points

- Polycystic ovary syndrome affects at least 10% of the female population.
- 20% of all females have polycystic ovaries on ultrasound scan and may be at risk of developing symptoms.
- The symptoms of PCOS include irregular or absent periods, acne, excess body hair, weight gain, and difficulty becoming pregnant.

Polycystic ovary syndrome (PCOS) is the name given to a condition resulting from an imbalance in sex hormone production. As a result of the hormonal imbalance, symptoms such as irregular periods, acne, excess facial and body hair, or scalp hair thinning may develop (Table 1.1). PCOS affects an estimated 10 per cent of premenopausal women although many women remain undiagnosed. A number of women may have PCOS but may not realize that this is the cause of their symptoms as it can be embarrassing going to see your doctor to complain about excess hair growth or mood swings. Some women may have infrequent or absent periods and may be relieved not to 'suffer' each month like their friends, so do not seek advice from their doctor about their periods. Some women are only diagnosed when they are being investigated for fertility problems. Some women may feel guilty about being overweight, are worried they will be told that it is their fault, and are therefore reluctant to go to their doctor about it.

Approximately 1 in 5 women of childbearing age have polycystic ovaries. This describes the appearance of the ovaries when they are seen on ultrasound scan. 'Polycystic' means multiple cysts, but in reality it refers to several tiny follicles below the surface of one or both ovaries (Fig. 1.1). In polycystic

Table 1.1 Occurrence of symptoms in women with PCOS

Women with PCOS may have one or more of the following:	
Irregular or absent periods	80%
Difficulty becoming pregnant	40%
Increased facial and body hair	70%
Acne and oily skin	20%
Thinning of scalp hair	15%
Weight gain and difficulty losing weight	50%

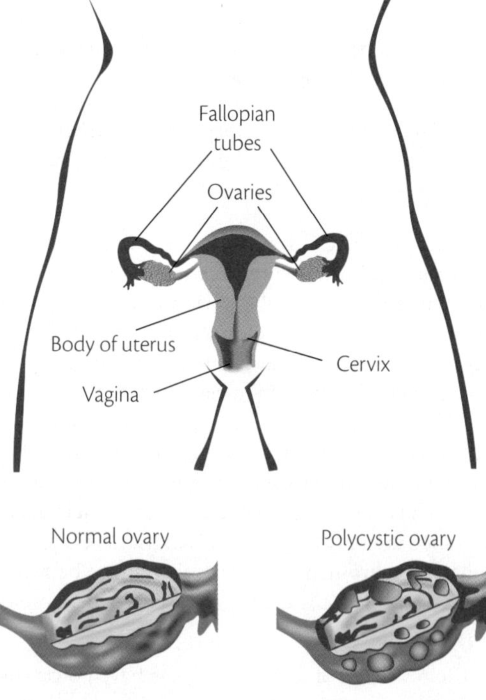

Figure 1.1 Normal versus polycystic ovaries.

ovaries, approximately twice as many follicles than usual will develop because of the hormonal disturbance, resulting in slightly larger than normal ovaries. PCOS is the name given to the condition in which women with polycystic ovaries have one or more symptoms (Table 1.1). One study showed that up to 80 per cent of women who had polycystic ovaries on ultrasound and who were previously thought to be asymptomatic actually had either irregular periods or unwanted hair.

Are these cysts harmful?

No. These cysts are only a few millimetres (<9 mm) in size, do not in themselves cause problems, and represent partially developed eggs that were not released. The word 'cyst' is misleading as what is seen on ultrasound are multiple tiny egg follicles. The follicles do not need surgery and are not associated with an increased risk of ovarian cancer. Removing the follicles will not improve any of the symptoms of PCOS.

2

What causes polycystic ovary syndrome?

Key points

- The exact cause of PCOS is unknown.
- Polycystic ovary syndrome tends to run in families and is more common in women with a family history of diabetes.
- The symptoms of PCOS are thought to be caused by an imbalance of the hormones controlling the menstrual cycle and an increase in insulin secretion, resulting in an increase in testosterone production by the ovaries.

In order for you to understand what happens in PCOS, it is important to understand the mechanism and control of the menstrual cycle and ovulation.

Women have two ovaries located in the pelvis on either side of the uterus (womb). Their main functions are to produce sex hormones and develop eggs. All of the eggs that you have throughout your life are made before you are born and are stored in the ovaries in an immature form. The eggs lie inactive until puberty, following which each month one egg is activated and matures in response to hormonal changes in the menstrual cycle. The ovaries produce three main hormones—oestrogen, progesterone ('female' hormones), and androgens ('male' hormones). The function of the ovaries is regulated by the pituitary gland which is a pea-sized gland located at the base of the brain just behind the bridge of your nose. It is often referred to as the 'master gland', because it releases hormones which regulate the function of the majority of the glands in the body. The pituitary gland produces follicle-stimulating hormone (FSH) and luteinizing hormone (LH). FSH stimulates the growth and maturation of the egg follicle and oestrogen production, whereas LH stimulates androgen production and triggers ovulation. The concentration of both hormones varies throughout the menstrual cycle, with an LH peak immediately before ovulation. The pituitary gland in turn is controlled by a part of the brain called the hypothalamus, which is situated immediately above the pituitary gland. The hypothalamus produces gonadotrophin-releasing hormone (GnRH) in a pulse-like manner which stimulates the release of FSH and LH, and ultimately controls menstruation and ovulation (Fig. 2.1). The function of the hypothalamus can be affected by weight—if you are too thin or too overweight this can affect the release of GnRH and thus affect your menstrual cycle. Severe stress or any severe illness can also switch this hormone off, resulting in missed or absent periods. This is the body's way of allowing pregnancy only when you are in good health.

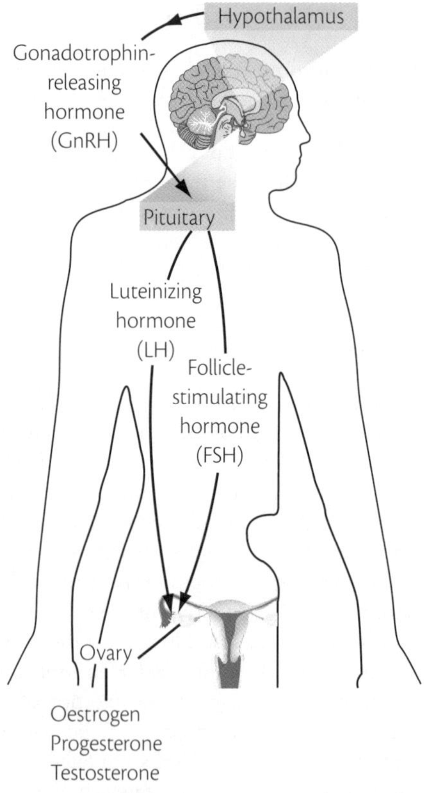

Figure 2.1 Hypothalamus, pituitary gland, and the ovaries and their hormones.

Puberty

Puberty is the term used to describe the physical and psychological changes that occur during the period of sexual maturation from childhood into adulthood. The first sign of puberty in females is usually the development of breasts, and normally starts between the ages of 8 and 13 years. The onset of puberty is determined by various hormonal changes. During childhood, the production of GnRH by the hypothalamus is 'switched off' and it is activated about 2 years before the onset of puberty. The production of GnRH will then stimulate FSH and LH secretion by the pituitary gland, which in turn will stimulate oestrogen and androgen production by the ovaries. The trigger for activating GnRH production and hence puberty is unclear, but we do know that it is dependent on genetic influences as well as nutritional factors. That is, girls have to reach a certain weight before puberty starts. Underweight girls tend to start puberty later and those who are overweight tend to start it at an earlier age. This may, at least in part, be due to increasing blood concentrations of a hormone known as leptin. Leptin is a protein produced by fat cells which has recently been shown to play an important role in reflecting the amount of body energy stores and thus triggering the onset of puberty. Other hormones that play a role in puberty include androgens produced by the adrenal glands, growth hormone, and insulin.

The menstrual cycle

Approximately 3 years after the onset of breast development, menstruation starts. Day 1 of the menstrual cycle is the first day of your period. During the menstrual cycle, 4–5 follicles, which are egg-containing fluid-filled sacs, will grow but usually only one follicle will mature—the dominant follicle—and the rest will degenerate. FSH secreted by the pituitary gland stimulates the growth of the egg follicles and also stimulates oestrogen production by the follicular cells surrounding the egg. Oestrogen also helps stimulate the egg in the follicle to grow and mature. Once the dominant follicle has a reached a size of at least 15 mm, its cells produce enough oestrogen to trigger a surge in production of LH by the pituitary gland (Figure 2.2a). This in turn triggers ovulation, whereby the dominant follicle bursts and releases its matured egg into the Fallopian tube. At the same time, oestrogen produced by the growing follicles stimulates the growth of the lining of the womb (endometrium) in preparation for pregnancy. If the egg is not fertilized, then the womb lining is shed about 14 days after ovulation, menstruation occurs, and the cycle then starts again. Progesterone is made following ovulation by the empty follicle, which is now known as the corpus luteum. Progesterone stops the release of more eggs and prepares the womb for implantation of a fertilized egg and pregnancy by stimulating the development of blood vessels in the lining of the womb. It can be measured in the latter half of the menstrual cycle as an indicator of ovulation. If pregnancy does not occur, the corpus luteum shrivels and the falling level of oestrogen and progesterone allows for complete shedding of the womb lining during menstruation. The first half of the menstrual cycle is known as the 'follicular phase' as the predominant feature is maturation of

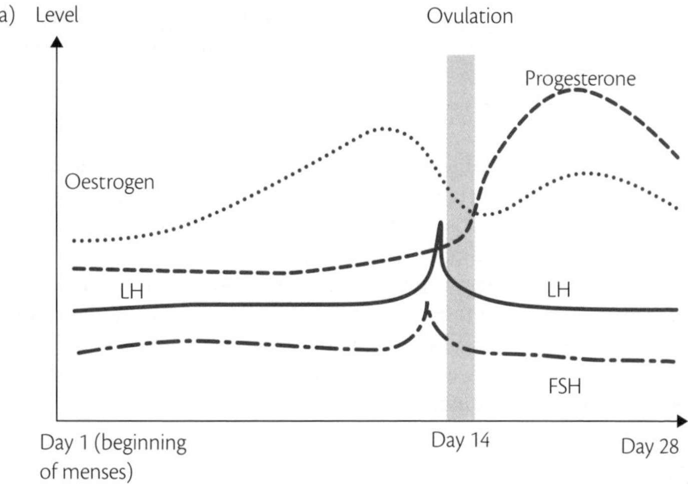

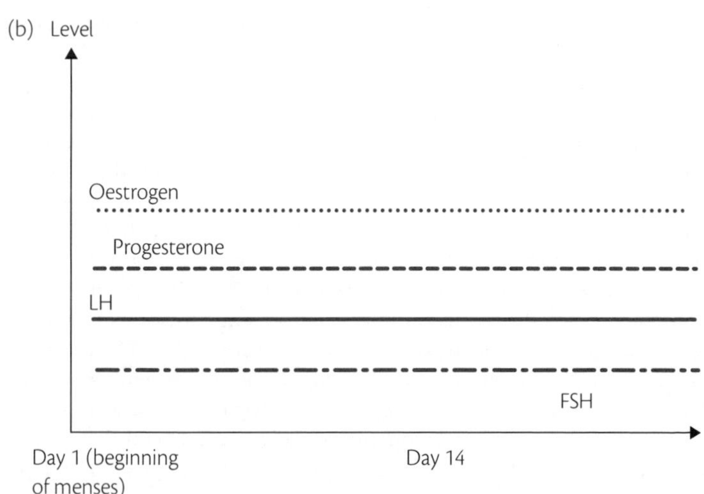

Figure 2.2 (a) Normal menstrual cycle and (b) the cycle in PCOS.

a follicle, and the second half of the cycle is know as the 'luteal' phase after the corpus luteum. Male hormones, particularly testosterone, are made by the cells surrounding the follicles. Testosterone is then taken up by the cells of the dominant follicle and converted to oestrogen. Small amounts of androgens are essential for normal egg development, but too much testosterone can adversely affect egg quality and prevent ovulation.

In PCOS . . .

The exact cause of PCOS is unknown. We know that in PCOS there are two fundamental disturbances—an imbalance in the amount of hormones produced by the ovaries, and insulin resistance. What triggers these abnormalities is unclear. There appears to be a genetic influence, with PCOS running in families and being more common in women with a family history of type 2 diabetes. Studies have shown that up to 40 per cent of women with PCOS have either an affected sister or mother, or have a close relative with diabetes. The exact genes responsible for PCOS are unknown but a lot of research is being carried out in this field. Genes that control insulin and sex hormone production and action, and genes that control weight are of particular interest. PCOS may be inherited from either parent. In men, it may manifest itself as premature balding (before the age of 30 years). It seems likely that in the future more than one gene will be identified which will determine a woman's likelihood of developing PCOS, the type of symptoms she will suffer from, and how severe the condition will be. Lifestyle factors and possibly stress are also important. For example, many women have very few symptoms until they put on weight, following which the symptoms become a lot worse.

The symptoms of PCOS are caused by an imbalance in the hormones controlling the menstrual cycle (Fig. 2.2b). Many women with PCOS have a persistently high LH concentration and a constant FSH level. The high LH levels often stimulate the ovaries to produce an increased amount of androgens, particularly testosterone. The hormonal changes can result in failure of the ovarian follicles to mature properly and so many small immature follicles are present, as seen on ultrasound. As a result, no egg is released, ovulation does not occur, and progesterone is not produced. Periods are then irregular or even absent. Women with PCOS usually produce enough oestrogen as some of the testosterone is converted to oestrogen in the immature follicles.

About 25 per cent of women with PCOS also produce a little too much male hormone, or androgens, in their adrenal glands. The adrenal glands lie just above the kidneys and produce hormones such as cortisol that are essential for life and for coping with stress. The adrenal glands also produce small amounts of androgens. Adrenal androgens are responsible for the growth of pubic hair during puberty and are also thought to play a role in maintaining general well-being in women. For example, deficiency of adrenal androgens can cause low libido and energy levels in women. However, excessive production can results in irregular periods, acne, and hairiness.

Insulin resistance and PCOS

As far back as 1921, two French doctors described the presence of diabetes in women with excessive facial hair. However, it was not until the 1980s that it was established that a high insulin level is a fundamental disturbance in most overweight women with PCOS and in about a third of slim women with PCOS. Insulin is a hormone released from the pancreas after a meal containing carbohydrates. Its main function is to control blood sugar levels. Insulin allows the liver and muscle cells to take up glucose (sugar) and use it as energy. Any excess glucose in the blood is converted into fat. In PCOS, the cells in the body do not use insulin efficiently, so to compensate the pancreas makes more insulin to try and move the sugar out of the blood and into the cells. This is known as 'insulin resistance'. If the pancreas cannot keep up with the increased demand, blood sugar will rise and diabetes develops. Insulin resistance can exacerbate excess weight gain as high insulin levels can be associated with sugar and carbohydrate cravings, resulting in overeating. Additionally, insulin resistance encourages the conversion of blood glucose to fat rather than being used as energy. Unfortunately, excess fat associated with weight gain makes the insulin resistance worse, resulting in a further rise in insulin levels, and a vicious circle develops. A sedentary lifestyle and high stress levels can also increase insulin resistance, making symptoms worse. Insulin resistance may also explain the reason why the symptoms of PCOS often develop during puberty. High insulin levels are a common finding in puberty as high levels of growth hormone, while necessary for growth, cause insulin resistance.

Insulin stimulates the ovarian cells to grow and produce sex hormones (Figure 2.3). In contrast to the rest of the body's cells in women with PCOS, the ovaries are not resistant to the effects of insulin and the excessively high levels stimulate the ovaries to produce more testosterone. Excess insulin and sex hormones also work together to stimulate the pituitary gland to secrete more LH, and the excess LH stimulates the ovary's testosterone production even more. Finally, the high levels of insulin reduce the production of a protein by the liver that binds testosterone in the blood—sex hormone-binding globulin (SHBG). This means that there is more free testosterone available to act on the skin.

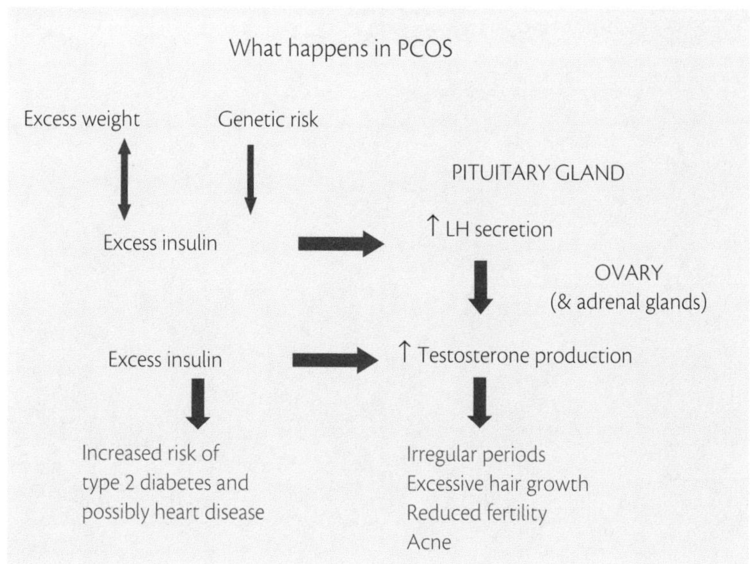

Figure 2.3 The role of insulin in PCOS.

History of PCOS

In 1935, Drs Stein and Leventhal described seven women who were very overweight, had no periods, and had excessive facial hair growth. At surgery these women were found to have large cystic ovaries, and so they named this condition 'polycystic ovarian disease', often since referred to as Stein–Leventhal syndrome. The diagnosis was initially only made in women with severe forms of the syndrome. In the 1960s and 1970s it was discovered that a lot of women with what is now known as PCOS have raised testosterone levels. In the 1980s it was discovered that up to 20 per cent of all women of childbearing age have polycystic ovaries on ultrasound, though only half of these women have symptoms and many women were only mildly affected. Also in the 1980s the association between insulin resistance, PCOS, and diabetes mellitus was increasingly recognized. Finally, over the past decade, a lot more has been learnt about the hereditary factors causing PCOS, the wide variation in symptoms, and the risks associated with PCOS. Learning more about PCOS through research enables us to find the most effective ways of controlling the symptoms and reducing the health risks associated with PCOS. Finally, it is hoped that one day research into PCOS may help us find a cure.

3

What are the symptoms of polycystic ovary syndrome?

Key points

- PCOS affects women in different ways, with some having severe symptoms whereas others may only be mildly affected.
- The symptoms of PCOS include irregular or absent periods, acne, excess body hair, weight gain, and difficulty becoming pregnant.

PCOS affects women in different ways, with some having severe symptoms whereas others may only be mildly affected. Symptoms often develop at the time of puberty or late teens, following weight gain or after coming off the contraceptive pill, but can occur at any time. If you have PCOS you may have some or all of the following symptoms.

Irregular periods

The normal menstrual cycle can vary from 21 to 35 days. Irregular or absent periods affect around 75 per cent of women with PCOS. The period disturbance is a sign that there is a problem with regular monthly ovulation. Oestrogen production by the follicles stimulates growth of the womb lining; however, if there is no ovulation, the lining is not shed and becomes abnormally thickened. This can lead to irregular, infrequent, and often very heavy periods. Eighty-five to ninety per cent of women who have periods more than 40 days apart are thought to have PCOS.

Reduced fertility

PCOS is a common cause of subfertility. Seventy to eighty per cent of women who fail to ovulate have PCOS. The cause of lack of ovulation is failure of the follicles to mature and release an egg each month. Irregular cycles or amenorrhoea (absent periods) usually indicate lack of or infrequent ovulation. However, some women with PCOS will ovulate normally and some will ovulate less frequently or will not ovulate at all. Some women will ovulate infrequently despite having 'regular' periods and only discover they have PCOS when being investigated for failure to conceive.

Miscarriage

Women with PCOS may also be at increased risk of miscarriage. The cause is unclear, but it is thought that the hormonal imbalance, particularly high LH and insulin levels, in PCOS may interfere with egg development and may disrupt embryo implantation within the womb. However, many women with PCOS are able to conceive and to carry successful pregnancies to term.

Increased hairiness (hirsutism)

Excess androgens produced by the ovaries and adrenal glands may enter the blood circulation and react with receptors on the skin, causing excessive hairiness. Many women with PCOS develop unwanted hair on their face, chest, tummy, arms, or legs. Hair that was previously light in colour and texture can be stimulated by testosterone, resulting in darkening and coarsening of hair in a male-pattern distribution.

Acne

Oil production in the skin is stimulated by testosterone. Women with PCOS may therefore complain of greasy spotty skin. Acne may develop on the face, chest, and/or back.

Frontal hair thinning

Occasionally excess testosterone can result in head hair thinning on the top of the head and at the temples.

The presence and degree of hairiness, acne, and frontal hair thinning vary according to your skin's sensitivity to the effects of androgens. Your genes and ethnic origin may influence this sensitivity to androgens. For example, women of Mediterranean or Asian origin tend to have a high skin sensitivity to androgens, whilst Oriental and Scandinavian women might not have any skin symptoms in spite of high androgen levels.

Weight gain or difficulty losing weight

Commonly a woman with PCOS will have what is called an apple figure where weight is concentrated heavily in the abdomen, with comparatively thinner arms and legs. Fat cells around and inside the tummy are particularly sensitive to the effects of insulin compared with those in the rest of the body. Insulin tends to prevent the breakdown of fat from the abdomen.

Approximately 50–60 per cent of women with PCOS are overweight, but even slimmer women with PCOS and insulin resistance find it difficult to lose fat from around their stomach. Excess weight often worsens the other symptoms of PCOS by increasing insulin resistance, which in turn increases ovarian sex hormone production. Unfortunately, the hormone changes associated with PCOS make weight loss more difficult. The reason for this is unclear. Certainly high insulin levels can increase your appetite, can give you carbohydrate cravings, and make it easier for you to store fat rather than burn it off. Many women with PCOS have low self-esteem as a result of the distressing symptoms, and another reason for excess weight gain is that depression and low self-esteem contribute to emotional eating and reluctance to exercise.

Other

Some women complain of **pelvic pain**. The cause of this is unclear. **Skin tags** can form and are usually found in the armpits or neck. These can easily be removed. Darkening and thickening of the skin can also occur around the neck, groin, underarms, or skin folds. This is known as **acanthosis nigricans**. Both skin tags and acanthosis nigricans are a sign of insulin resistance. If you have PCOS you may also suffer from **mood swings** or **unexplained fatigue**.

Some rarer hormonal conditions can cause insulin resistance or excess androgen production, and may result in polycystic ovaries on ultrasound and symptoms similar to PCOS. These conditions should be excluded first before being treated for PCOS. Your doctor will arrange the appropriate tests if he/she is concerned.

4

What are the health risks associated with polycystic ovary syndrome?

Key points

- Having PCOS may increase the risk of developing diabetes, abnormal blood fats, high blood pressure, and possibly heart disease.
- Eating healthily and controlling your weight may reduce the health risks associated with PCOS
- Women with PCOS who have no periods at all may also be at increased risk of cancer of the lining of the womb. This is a rare complication of PCOS and the risk can be minimized by medication.

It is becoming increasingly apparent that women with PCOS, particularly if they are overweight, are at increased risk of developing certain conditions (Figure 4.1). This chapter summarizes the health risks associated with having PCOS and discusses how to minimize the risks.

Metabolic syndrome and diabetes

Metabolic syndrome is a term describing a constellation of abnormalities associated with insulin resistance. It describes the presence of central obesity (weight gain around the waist) and at least two of the following: diabetes or abnormal glucose tolerance ('pre-diabetes'), high blood pressure, and abnormal blood fats. Overweight women with PCOS are at increased risk of developing the metabolic syndrome, and its presence increases the risk of developing heart disease and diabetes.

Type 2 diabetes (non-insulin dependent) occurs when the pancreas is unable to keep producing excess insulin to maintain normal blood sugar levels. One study in menopausal women who had been treated for PCOS 30 years earlier showed they were seven times more likely to have diabetes. Studies indicate that up to a third of overweight women with PCOS will develop glucose intolerance and 10 per cent will develop diabetes by the age of 40 years. These rates are much higher than expected for women at this young age. The risk of developing diabetes is highest in overweight women but is also increased in slim women with PCOS who are insulin resistant. The risk of developing diabetes is increased further in women with a family history of diabetes. However, studies have shown that you can more than halve your risk of developing diabetes by healthy eating, increasing physical activity, and weight loss if you are overweight. The Royal College of Obstetrics and Gynaecology recommends that women with PCOS are screened regularly for the presence of diabetes as symptoms are often absent. However, experts are still unsure about at what age to start screening, how best to screen, and how often the tests need to be done. We currently screen all women at the time of diagnosis with a fasting blood sugar and occasionally a glucose tolerance test. If the test is normal, then we would repeat this every year in overweight women and every 3 years in women of normal body weight.

Women with PCOS and insulin resistance are also more likely to develop **high blood pressure** as they become older. High blood pressure (hypertension) rarely makes people feel ill, and often the only way of knowing if you have hypertension is to have your blood pressure measured. People with high blood pressure run a higher risk of having a stroke or a heart attack, but reducing your blood pressure can lower your risk of developing any of these problems. For some overweight women, losing weight is all they need to do to get their blood pressure down. Becoming more physically active, reducing salt intake, and increasing the amount of fruit and vegetables in your diet all help to control blood pressure.

Finally, women with PCOS, particularly if overweight, are more likely to develop **abnormal blood fats** (lipids). There are two main blood fats in the body: cholesterol and triglycerides. Cholesterol is a fatty substance which is mainly made by the liver from saturated fats in food. It plays an important role in cell function, but too much cholesterol in the blood can increase the risk of developing heart disease. Cholesterol is transported in the bloodstream attached to proteins, the combination of which is known as 'lipoproteins'. There are two main lipoproteins—low-density lipoproteins (LDLs), which carry cholesterol from the liver to the cells, and high-density lipoproteins (HDLs), which remove cholesterol from the circulation and appear to protect against coronary heart disease. Overweight women with PCOS are more likely to have low levels of

HDL-cholesterol and high triglyceride levels, increasing the risk of developing heart disease. Some women with PCOS may also have higher LDL-cholesterol levels compared with other women of the same age.

Increasing physical activity can increase your HDL-cholesterol, reducing your risk of heart disease. Shedding pounds if you are overweight can also reduce triglyceride and increase HDL-cholesterol levels.

Gestational diabetes

Women with PCOS who become pregnant, especially if overweight, are at risk of developing gestational diabetes, or diabetes of pregnancy. It is therefore advisable that you be screened at 12 weeks of pregnancy for diabetes. If the test is normal then you should be tested again for gestational diabetes at 28 and 32 weeks of pregnancy. This form of diabetes tends to go away after delivery but does indicate that you are at risk of developing type 2 diabetes later in life. You should therefore have a blood sugar check yearly following a diagnosis of gestational diabetes. By eating healthily, exercising, and losing weight if you are overweight you can significantly reduce your risk of developing diabetes.

Heart disease

It is becoming more evident that women with PCOS may be at increased risk of developing coronary heart disease, particularly after the menopause. Several studies showed that middle-aged women with PCOS were more likely to have narrowed coronary arteries (blood vessels supplying the heart) compared with other women of similar age. The Nurses' Health Study followed over 100 000 women for over 8 years and found that women who had irregular periods in early adulthood, the most common cause being PCOS, were one and a half times more likely to develop heart disease than women with regular periods. Other factors that increase the risk of heart disease are summarized in table 4.1.

How to reduce your risk of heart disease

1. Eat healthily

   Try to eat a diet low in saturated fats and try to avoid processed foods. Try to eat at least five portions of fruit and vegetables a day. See Chapter 14 for further advice.

2. Become more physically active

   Research has shown that a sedentary lifestyle doubles the risk of developing heart disease even in women with normal body weight.

Table 4.1 Known risk factors for heart disease

Male sex
Increasing age (risk increases significantly after the menopause in women)
Family history
Diabetes
High blood pressure
Cigarette smoking
High LDL- and low HDL-cholesterol levels
High blood triglyceride levels
Obesity
Physical inactivity

3. Lose weight if you are overweight

   Studies have shown a significantly increased risk of heart disease in overweight men and women. By losing weight you can reduce your risk of developing heart disease.

4. Stop smoking

   Do see your doctor to discuss ways in which he/she can help you to stop smoking.

5. Ensure diabetes, high blood pressure, and/or abnormal blood fats are under control

An improvement may be achieved by lifestyle modification alone, but medication is often necessary to optimize control. Do attend your clinic appointments with your doctor or nurse so they can keep an eye on your progress and ensure you are on the appropriate treatment.

Endometrial cancer

Women with PCOS who do not have periods for a long time, particularly if they are overweight, appear to be at slightly increased risk of developing cancer of the lining of the womb (endometrial cancer) if the lack of periods is not treated. This is because oestrogens stimulate the womb lining to grow but the

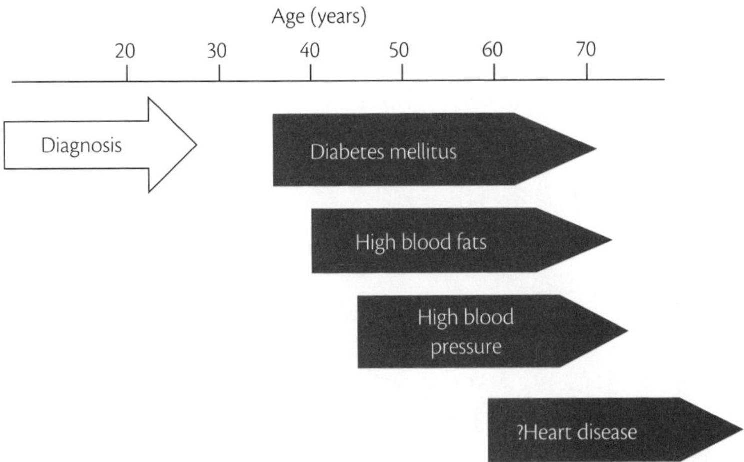

Figure 4.1 Health risks associated with PCOS.

lack of ovulation means that progesterone is not produced and efficient shedding does not occur. The thickness of the endometrium can be measured using an internal ultrasound and, if necessary, a biopsy can be taken. Fortunately, this cancer is rare and the risk can be minimized by inducing 4–5 periods a year using medication. By eating healthily and undertaking regular exercise you can improve your hormonal imbalance and, by so doing, you may be able to regulate your periods naturally.

There is no evidence at the moment to suggest that PCOS *per se* increases the risk of other cancers. However, we do know that obesity does increase the risk of certain cancers such as breast cancer.

Although having PCOS increases the risk of developing certain diseases, the good news is that a recent study indicates that women with PCOS have a completely normal life expectancy. In addition, the health risks can be minimized significantly by adopting a healthier lifestyle. Improving your diet, increasing your physical activity, and losing weight if you are carrying extra weight will all go some way towards preventing heart disease and diabetes, and may also improve some of the symptoms associated with PCOS.

5

How is the diagnosis of polycystic ovary syndrome made?

Key points

- The diagnosis of PCOS is made on the basis of a combination of clinical observation and the results of investigations.
- The diagnosis is made in the presence of at least two of the following: evidence of excess testosterone production, irregular periods, and/or polycystic ovaries on ultrasound
- There is no cure for PCOS but a lot can be done to control the symptoms and reduce the health risks.

There has been a lot of discussion among doctors about how best to diagnose PCOS, particularly since the symptoms of PCOS can be very variable. European doctors put a lot of emphasis on the ultrasound findings, whereas in the USA more emphasis was put on period and skin problems. However, in 2003, PCOS specialists from Europe and America met and agreed that PCOS was present if at least two of the following criteria were met:

- Presence of excess androgens, either on blood testing or as evidenced by symptoms such as excess body hair, acne, or male pattern hair thinning
- Irregular or absent periods
- Presence of polycystic ovaries on ultrasound
- After the exclusion of other medical conditions that can result in the above.

Investigations your doctor may ask for to help make the diagnosis include the following.

Ultrasound scan

This is usually done as an internal scan, meaning that a small ultrasound probe is placed just inside the vagina, giving the best views of the ovaries and pelvic organs. Some of you may not feel comfortable with an internal scan, for example if you are still a virgin. In that case an external scan performed over your lower tummy can be done. To get good pictures of your ovaries using an external scan, you will need to have a full bladder so you will be asked to drink a lot of water just before the scan.

In PCOS, one or both ovaries are enlarged and have 12 or more small cysts (follicles) around the edge, resulting in a 'string of pearls' appearance (Fig. 5.1). This is a result of the hormonal disturbance rather than the cause of symptoms. A PCOS diagnosis cannot be made entirely on the basis of ultrasound alone as not all women with PCOS have this typical appearance of their ovaries on ultrasound scan. Conversely, not all women with polycystic ovaries have symptoms. However, polycystic ovaries on ultrasound indicate that a woman is at risk of developing symptoms and thus PCOS at a later stage in her life, for example if she puts on too much weight. Finally, causes of male hormone excess or insulin resistance other than PCOS can result in polycystic ovaries on ultrasound although fortunately these are extremely uncommon. The internal scan can also be used to measure the thickness of the womb lining (endometrium) to assess whether it is overgrown or not in women with

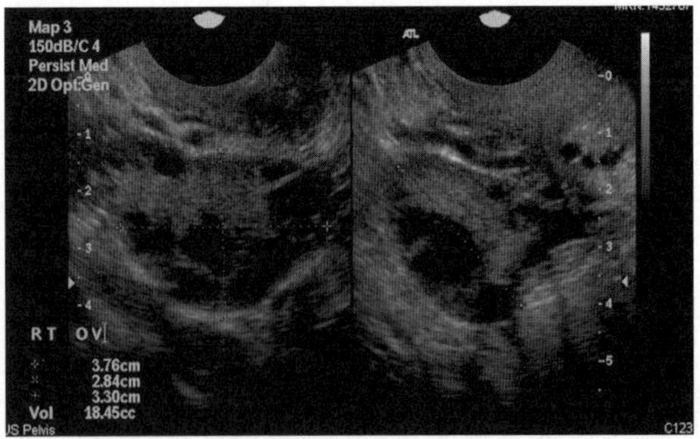

Figure 5.1 Ultrasound appearance of PCOS.

absent or infrequent periods, and this will determine whether treatment for the irregular periods is necessary.

Blood tests

Your doctor may ask for blood tests to help make the diagnosis (Table 5.1). He/she may want to check the level of androgens (male hormones), such as testosterone, and may also measure the hormones involved in ovulation—FSH and LH. If you are having periods, then the tests should be done in the first week of your menstrual cycle. The tests cannot be done while you are on the contraceptive pill as this will affect the results. You may have a high blood testosterone level; however, many of you may have been told that your testosterone level is normal. Women with PCOS are often very sensitive to testosterone, so even if the blood levels are normal symptoms of PCOS can develop. Your doctor may also arrange some tests to exclude diabetes and

Table 5.1 Investigation of PCOS

To make diagnosis	Notes
Ovarian ultrasound	Polycystic ovaries in 80–96%
Blood testosterone	High in 50–80%
Blood LH	High in 50–70%
Other investigations	
Blood FSH	Usually normal or slightly low
SHBG (sex hormone-binding globulin)	Usually low in insulin resistance
Thyroid function	Especially if fatigued, in the presence of weight gain, or irregular periods
Prolactin levels	Hormone produced by the pituitary gland. May be high in PCOS and may be associated with absent or irregular periods. If very high, then a scan of the pituitary gland may be recommended
Kidney and liver function	Before starting medication. Liver function tests may be abnormal in women who are obese as fat is deposited in the liver
Fasting glucose and lipids (blood fats)	To exclude diabetes and high fat levels
Fasting insulin levels or glucose tolerance test with insulin measurements	Some doctors may ask for this to diagnose insulin resistance

abnormal blood lipid (fat) levels and to look for evidence of insulin resistance. Finally, before drug treatment is started, a blood test to assess liver and kidney function is usually necessary. If you have some symptoms that may be caused by other conditions then your doctor may ask for more tests, for example thyroid function tests.

The diagnosis of PCOS is made on the basis of a combination of clinical observation and the results of investigations.

Your own GP can do the initial blood tests and may be able to arrange an ultrasound scan. Once the diagnosis is made, nothing more needs to be done for some women, for example if your weight is within normal limits, if you do not have excess body hair or acne, if you have at least one period every 3 months, and if you do not want to become pregnant. If any of the symptoms are an issue, then a specialist referral is needed for further advice and treatment.

Is there a cure for PCOS?

No, there is no cure, but there is a lot that you can do to help yourself. With the right medical support, some changes to what you eat and increasing your physical activity, you can manage some of the symptoms of PCOS and give yourself a much better chance of a healthy life. If you are overweight or have a family history of diabetes or heart disease, then it is particularly important that you look at ways of improving your lifestyle to reduce your risk of developing diabetes and possibly heart disease.

Medical treatment can certainly help control the symptoms of PCOS. If you have several symptoms then you and your doctor need to decide which symptom takes priority and the management plan can then be drawn up to target that particular symptom. For example, if you want to become pregnant but are also concerned about facial hair growth, then you may decide to try to conceive first as you cannot take medication to reduce your excess hair growth whilst trying for a baby.

Tips for your first appointment with your doctor

- Don't be afraid or embarrassed to go to your doctor. Doctors have seen so many women with symptoms similar to your own and will hopefully be able to help you understand and manage your symptoms. Ask to see a female doctor if that will make you feel more comfortable.

- Your GP should be able to talk through any concerns you may have, request the initial investigations, and explain the reasons behind his/her decision to refer you to the hospital specialist. You may be referred to a gynaecologist if your main problems are related to fertility or heavy periods, or you may be referred to an endocrinologist (hormone specialist) if your main problems are related to weight gain, skin complaints, or irregular periods.

- It can be daunting going to the hospital for the first time, and you might find it helpful if a close relative or friend goes with you so that they can offer support. Additionally, you tend to forget a certain percentage of what has been said, so having another person with you as another pair of ears will help you remember the key points.
- Go prepared. Doctors prepare to see you by checking any previous notes and results and reading information given by your GP before calling you in. The time spent with your doctor is usually limited, and therefore it is just as important for you to prepare so that you get the best from your visit. Before your appointment write down a list of your symptoms. It is sometimes hard to know which of your symptoms are significant, but it is best to give your doctor as much information as possible and then let him/her decide which symptoms merit further investigation or treatment.
- Bring a list of questions with you. You may find that many of your questions are answered throughout the course of the consultation. However, do ask any remaining questions at the end.
- Take a notepad and pen with you to write down important information your doctor gives you.
- Ask your doctor to explain anything you don't understand. It is important that you leave the clinic with a clear idea of your condition and treatment plan. Ask your doctor about success rates and side effects of the various treatment options, and ask if they have information leaflets on the options. You can then make an informed choice based on the information given to you and guidance from your doctor.
- When any medication is prescribed, make sure you receive full instructions on when and how to take it and enquire about any side effects you may experience.
- Finally, if you are not happy with your doctor's advice, you can ask for a second opinion.

Part 2

The treatment of polycystic ovary syndrome

6

Controlling insulin resistance

Key points

- Insulin resistance, present in at least half of all women with PCOS, indicates that the body is not using insulin efficiently and to compensate produces higher than usual levels of insulin.
- The presence of insulin resistance increases the risk of diabetes and possibly heart disease.
- Insulin resistance may be improved by eating healthily, being physically active, and losing weight if you are overweight. Metformin may also be used in some women to increase insulin sensitivity.

Insulin resistance plays an important role in the development of symptoms associated with PCOS and also increases the risk of developing diabetes, high blood pressure, abnormal blood fats, and heart disease (Chapter 4). If you have PCOS and insulin resistance then you are up to seven times more likely to develop diabetes than other women your age, particularly if you are overweight. Now, insulin resistance cannot be cured, but you can improve your insulin sensitivity by adopting a healthy lifestyle. At least three major studies showed that people who were at high risk of developing diabetes and who intensively improved their lifestyle more than halved their risk of developing diabetes. Studies have also shown that fertility in PCOS can be greatly enhanced and periods regulated by improving insulin sensitivity. This chapter will explain how you can do this.

What you can do

Diet

Lose weight if you are overweight. Studies have consistently shown that 5–10 per cent weight loss in overweight or obese women with PCOS can improve your body's response to insulin and significantly reduce your blood testosterone levels, while increasing your SHBG levels. This means there will be less free testosterone in your blood to act on your skin and ovaries, leading to an improvement in your symptoms. As little as 5 per cent weight loss, that is 10 lb if you weigh 200 lb, can significantly improve ovulation and your chances of pregnancy.

To lose weight safely and effectively aim for a 1/2 to 2 lb weight loss per week. Please see Part 3 for a detailed guide.

If you are not overweight, then you should still adopt a healthy diet in order to improve your insulin sensitivity and reduce your long-term health risks, although you obviously do not need to cut down on your daily caloric intake. As previously discussed, up to a third of slim women with PCOS are insulin resistant, and this is more likely if you have absent or irregular periods. By improving your diet you may be able to improve your menstrual cycle and enhance your fertility. Avoid specific foods that rapidly elevate blood glucose levels as high blood glucose levels are the trigger for the secretion of insulin. Foods with a high glycaemic index (GI) stimulate the release of insulin more than those with a low GI. By eating low- and medium-GI foods and eating enough protein with each meal (see Chapter 18), you will reduce your average insulin levels and hopefully improve your symptoms.

Exercise

Regular exercise (both aerobic and strength training) increases your cells' sensitivity to insulin. One study showed that walking briskly for 1 hour a day four times a week can result in a fall in insulin resistance by up to 25 per cent in women with PCOS. Even if you exercise and do not lose weight, you are still improving your insulin sensitivity and thus improving your health. It is important that you develop an exercise programme that you find enjoyable and can fit into your busy life, otherwise you will be unlikely to continue with it (see Chapter 16).

Stop smoking

Insulin resistance is worsened by nicotine and, as you probably already know, smoking increases your risk of developing heart disease and various cancers. Do seek the advice of your doctor if you are finding giving up smoking difficult. Different methods work for different people, so do discuss the available options with your nurse or doctor. Many surgeries run smoking cessation clinics to provide support and help to encourage you to stop smoking as we all know how difficult it is to give up.

Reduce your stress levels

We all feel stressed at various times in our lives. It is a normal response to certain life events, whether good or bad. Stress energizes us to cope with challenging circumstances, but being overstressed can result in a range of health problems. You cannot avoid stress entirely, but you can learn techniques to minimize the effects of stress on your body. Stress and inadequate sleep increase hormones such as cortisol and adrenaline which increase insulin resistance. Again, your goal is to reduce your already high insulin levels so try to reduce stress, for example by relaxation exercises, aromatherapy, or herbal remedies, if necessary, and try to go to bed at a reasonable hour (see Chapter 7).

Nutritional supplements

Very little research has been done looking at the use of nutritional supplements to treat insulin resistance and PCOS. However, it is known that chromium, zinc, and magnesium are all minerals involved in the regulation of insulin production and insulin sensitivity (Table 6.1). All may help control cravings and reduce hunger. Cinnamon may improve your body's response to insulin. Sprinkle 1/2–1 teaspoonful of cinnamon on your cereal every morning! The essential fatty acids, particularly omega-3 fatty acids, can also reduce insulin levels. Try to eat 2–3 portions of oily fish a week to increase your consumption of omega-3. If you have a balanced and healthy diet, then you should not need any additional supplements. However, modern diets do not always contain sufficient amounts of minerals. If you choose to take supplements, then we recommend that you see a medical nutritionist who can assess your diet and then prescribe supplements based on your needs. There are a vast number of vitamin and mineral preparations on the market but not all are of good quality—some are poorly absorbed and therefore a waste of money, whereas others may actually be harmful. Buy fish oil only from reputable companies to ensure that the product is free from chemical contamination and peroxides. Your medical nutritionist should be able to advise you on the best preparations. He/she can also advise you on which preparations are safe to take while trying to conceive. For example, fish oils and chromium supplements are not recommended during pregnancy. It is important that you see a reputable nutritionist, someone who is recommended by a friend or someone who is registered with a professional body.

Table 6.1 Minerals which may help reduce insulin resistance

Mineral	**Food rich in the mineral**	**Possible daily supplementation**
Chromium	Cheese, wholegrain cereals, brewer's yeast	200–400 mcg
Magnesium	Pulses, brown rice, green leafy vegetables, bananas and nuts, dried fruit	150–300 mg
Zinc	Seafood, parsley, chicken, sunflower seeds, mushrooms, eggs, oats and whole grain cereals	15 mg
Omega-3 fatty acid	Oily fish, e.g. mackerel, tuna, salmon	2 g

What your doctor can do

Metformin

Metformin is a drug that has been used in the treatment of diabetes for over 30 years. It is an 'insulin sensitizer', that is it acts by making the cells use insulin more efficiently. By doing so, the pancreas does not need to produce as much insulin and so there is less insulin to act on the ovaries. An extensive review of studies looking at the use of metformin in women with PCOS concluded that it significantly reduces insulin levels by improving the body's response to insulin. Several studies show that metformin can reduce blood androgen levels, make periods more regular and improving fertility in women with PCOS. If metformin alone does not restore ovulation, it may improve a woman's response to fertility drugs. The use of metformin may also make weight loss easier by improving insulin sensitivity and reducing carbohydrate cravings. Certainly in our clinic women who are able to take metformin appear to lose weight more successfully than those who do not. Metformin may, in addition, help reduce excess hair growth in insulin-resistant women with PCOS. Finally, there have recently been a couple of studies published which indicate that the use of metformin may reduce the risk of miscarriage in insulin-resistant women with PCOS. However, more research is needed before metformin is used routinely in pregnancy.

The effects on menstruation and ovulation can be seen as early as 3 months after starting treatment, but the effects on excess hair growth may not be evident for several months. However, do remember that there is no drug that is guaranteed to work in every woman. If, after 6 months of use, no beneficial effect has been seen, then there is no point in continuing metformin. If it is effective, then the duration of treatment will depend on the severity of your hormonal imbalance and whether or not it can be controlled with diet and exercise alone. If you are overweight, then we tend to treat you until you have reached your target weight, and then try and control your weight and other symptoms by diet and exercise alone. However, some of you may need to continue metformin on a long-term basis if your symptoms return when it is stopped. There do not appear to be any health risks from the prolonged use of metformin.

Are there any side effects?

Metformin can cause nausea, abdominal bloating, and flatulence. In severe cases, it can cause vomiting or diarrhoea. Most women tolerate it very well, particularly if the dose is increased gradually. To minimize side effects, the tablets should be taken in the middle of a meal or straight after a meal. Side effects usually settle after 1–2 weeks. If side effects persist, then the dose of metformin may have to be reduced and, in some cases, it may have to be stopped.

Since metformin does not stimulate production of insulin, it should not cause hypoglycaemia. Women with kidney failure or severe liver disease should not take metformin as this will increase the risk of a very rare but dangerous side effect called lactic acidosis. Your doctor should arrange a blood test to check your kidney and liver function before prescribing this drug for you. You should stop metformin temporarily the day of and for 48 h after an X-ray where an intravenous dye is administered as this can occasionally be associated with kidney problems. Metformin has been used in the treatment of diabetes for over 30 years and has not been associated with any other side effects. However, metformin is only licensed for the treatment of diabetes, not PCOS. Metformin is not an experimental drug, but its use in PCOS is relatively new.

Is metformin safe in pregnancy?

There are no known reports of abnormal babies in women who conceived whilst taking metformin or who continued metformin throughout pregnancy. However, it is still too early to recommend the routine continuation of metformin throughout pregnancy. Our recommendation is to stop it when pregnancy is confirmed.

Starting metformin

Quick route

500 mg a day for 1 week	then
500 mg twice a day for 1 week	then
500 mg three times a day for 1 week	then
1 g twice a day thereafter	

Do not increase the dose if side effects develop—wait until they have settled first.

Slow route (in women with side effects)

Week 1	250 mg once a day
Week 2	250 mg twice a day
Week 3	250 mg three times a day
Week 4	500 mg twice a day
Week 5	500mg three times a day
Week 6	1 g twice a day

Higher doses (up to 3 g a day) may be required if your BMI (body mass index) is over 38. The minimum effective dose is thought to be 500 mg three times a day. If side effects prevent you from reaching that dose, then you can ask your doctor for the 'slow release' version of metformin which appears less likely to cause side effects.

Patient's perspective

Emma, aged 25 years, decided to stop the contraceptive pill as she was convinced it was the cause of her weight gain. However, she became increasingly despondent as despite trying hard to lose weight she was unable to do so. One factor stopping her was that she felt hungry in between meals and craved chocolate. Furthermore, she had not had a period for 7 months and had developed acne on her face and back which she found distressing.

When Emma was seen at clinic she weighed 91 kg (14 stone 7 lb) and had a body mass index of 34. The low-GI diet was recommended and discussed, she was encouraged to increase her physical activity, and she was prescribed metformin. Six months later Emma reported that she was having far fewer chocolate cravings. She had been going to the gym three times a week and was walking to and from work. Emma had lost 10 kg (24 lb) and had had three periods. Her acne was better. Following 12 months of treatment, Emma weighed 76 kg (11 stone 7 lb), she had a BMI of 27, her periods occurred every 4 weeks, and her skin was completely clear.

Future

Other insulin-sensitizing drugs such as pioglitazone and rosiglitazone also improve the body's sensitivity to insulin and are currently being investigated for the treatment of insulin resistance in PCOS, with very encouraging results. They certainly reduce insulin and testosterone levels and improve ovulation. However, as they are relatively new drugs their safety during pregnancy is unknown. Additionally, they can cause some weight gain, already a problem for many of you!

7

Coping with stress

 Key points

- Stress occurs when you feel unable to cope with the demands being put on you.
- Prolonged stress is both emotionally and physically exhausting and is associated with an increased susceptibility to certain illnesses.
- To reduce stress you need to identify the cause and investigate ways of minimizing its effect on you.

Stress occurs when you perceive that you cannot handle the demands put on you. We all develop stress at some stage in our lives in response to both positive and negative life events. A little bit of pressure is actually a good thing as it motivates us, enhances our performance, and makes us focus on the tasks ahead (Fig. 7.1). You have often heard people talk about 'performing under pressure'. However, too much pressure can lead to stress which can be both physically and emotionally exhausting. When our body is stressed, it releases hormones such as cortisol and adrenaline which help us survive by making us able to fight harder or run away from danger. This is known as the 'fight or flight response'. High levels of these hormones over a period of time, however, can affect our ability to think clearly and therefore may harm our work performance and our relationships (Fig. 7.1). If stress is prolonged, then these hormones may also increase our risk of developing heart disease, high blood pressure, and stroke, as well as other conditions. Persistent stress can also affect our immune system, making us more vulnerable to colds and other infections. Finally, persistently high levels of cortisol and adrenaline can result in an increase in the body's resistance to insulin, exacerbating symptoms associated with PCOS. For example, you may find that during stressful periods of your life your periods may become erratic or stop completely.

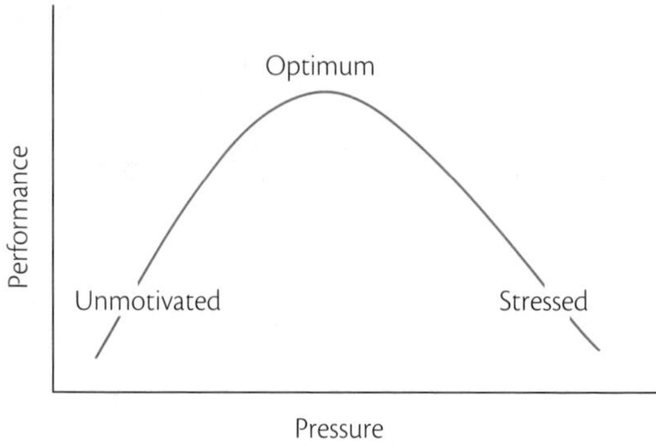

Figure 7.1 Stress–performance curve.

To reduce stress, you need first to identify that you are stressed by being aware of the symptoms of stress (Table 7.1). Can you identify with any of these feelings?

> I don't have time for myself anymore.
>
> I have difficulty sleeping.
>
> I get regular headaches.
>
> I am finding it difficult to cope.
>
> I open a bottle of wine when I get home from work to relax.

If so, then you may be stressed. This chapter will provide you with a general guide to relieving stress and minimize its affect on your health. What will work for one person may not be the answer for someone else, and so you will need to find the most suitable method for you.

What causes stress?

Different things trigger stress in different people. Stress can be caused by a whole range of pressures. Examples are:

- Conflict in relationships either at home or at work
- Feeling that you are not valued by others or that you have little support from colleagues, friends, or family members
- Change of social circumstances such as death of a loved one or unemployment, but positive changes such as marriage or moving home may also increase stress

Table 7.1 Stress symptoms checklist

Physical signs	Mental signs
Headaches	Indecision
Palpitations	Loss of concentration
Tiredness	Making mistakes
Muscle aches or pains	Worrying
Skin rashes	Depressed
Excessive sweating	Irritability
Frequent colds or other infections	Persistent negative thoughts
Lump in throat	Withdrawn
Dry mouth	Feeling tense, anxious, apprehensive
Loss of appetite or overeating	No enthusiasm, drained
Sweaty palms	Poor sleep
Tremulousness	Drinking more alcohol and/or smoking more
Diarrhoea	

- Too many simultaneous demands from different people at work and/or at home
- High-pressure job with a large volume of work and tight deadlines.

The degree of stress caused by these factors often varies according to individuals. We all cope differently with stress and some of us are able to tolerate a lot more than others.

Identify the cause of your stress

Keep a diary. Record the following:

- How stressed you are feeling
- What symptoms you are feeling
- What is causing you to be stressed
- How you respond to the stressful event and whether your reaction improves the situation or makes it worse.

By analysing your diary you will become aware of the warning symptoms and signs and gain a clearer understanding of the situations causing you most stress. You can then try and work out ways to minimize the stressful event.

Stress management

- Are you able to remove the cause of your stress?
    - If you only treat the symptoms of stress, for example taking pain killers to reduce muscle aches, the stress remains and the aches will return. If you are able to remove the cause of stress, then the muscle aches will disappear altogether.
    - Try to be detached when you look at the issues that are causing you to be stressed and try to come up with as many solutions as you can. You may be able to relieve it completely or at least reduce the level of stress. For example, if you are working very long hours in order to meet tight deadlines, are you able to delegate some of the work? If you are finding it difficult to juggle work with the demands of family life, are you able to get help with childcare or housework?
    - Are you able to take 'time out' from the stressful event? For example, if you are getting very upset or angry, can you leave the room and go for a walk? If work is quite pressurized, are you able to book a holiday?
    - One of the most important factors in reducing stress levels is managing time effectively (Table 7.2). You may need to list the tasks you want to do and prioritize them so that you are not trying to do everything at once. Try to be realistic about what you are able to achieve in a given time period.
    - Try to minimize the impact of stress on an event by preparing for it. For example, if you study for an exam or rehearse before giving a talk you will feel less anxious.
    - Understand and accept that there are certain things you will be unable to change. Instead, try to adjust your response and adapt to the situation.
- Try to change your mental approach to stressful events. The way we think has a direct effect on how we feel and how we behave. Often it is the way we perceive the situation that results in us feeling stressed. We are often over-critical of ourselves, and feel that we are doomed for failure. These types of negative thoughts can damage our confidence and harm our performance.
    - Try to take a step back and look at the situation as if it is happening to someone else. How would you advise them? It is usually easier to offer rational advice when you are detached from the situation.

Table 7.2 Time management

• Prioritize the demands on your time regularly so that you tackle urgent or important tasks first
• Always delegate tasks which can be done by someone else
• Keep a diary of your working day for a couple of weeks and try to analyse it to see where time is being 'wasted', for example several interruptions, reading irrelevant e-mails, or browsing unhelpful websites. You may then be able to think of ways of avoiding unproductive tasks and using your time more effectively
• List your short-term and long-term goals but be realistic about what you can achieve
• Try to put aside some time for yourself every day to collect your thoughts, assess priorities, and relax
• Learn to say no, so that you do not take on more than you can handle and you are not wasting time doing something that you consider low priority

- Believe in yourself. You wouldn't have been given the job if you didn't have the ability to do it.
- Set realistic goals and expectations for yourself and then try to minimize negative thinking.
- Try not to over-react—if a meeting did not go how you had planned it, then that does not mean that you are a failure.

- Try not to dwell on the negatives of a situation but focus on the positives.
- Do recognize your achievements and do not expect things to go right 100 per cent of the time. If things go wrong then do not be too harsh on yourself—learn from your mistakes but do try not to blow things out of all proportion.
- Worrying about the past or the future does not help, so try so concentrate on your next task. Try not to let worries dominate your day.
- Try not to blame yourself for all things that go wrong.
- Minimizing negative thoughts and substituting them with more positive and realistic ones will not happen overnight but, by attempting to change the way you interpret stressful situations, it will get easier and you will feel less stressed over time.

- Manage your physical response to stress
    - Relaxation techniques—breathe in slowly and deeply and count to 5 then breathe out slowly and count to 5, lowering your shoulders as you do so. Pause, and then repeat this slow breathing until you feel more relaxed. Stretch your muscles: for example, turn your neck to the left as far as it will go, hold for 5 seconds, and then relax. Turn your neck to the right, hold for 5 seconds, and relax. Pull your shoulders back, hold for 5 seconds and relax, then shrug your shoulders, hold the position for about 5 seconds, and then relax.
    - Work off stress by exercising. Do try and fit in some regular exercise in your day, even if it is just a short walk. Physical activity releases 'feel good' hormones called endorphins and reduces the level of stress hormones. Exercise also distracts us from the stressful situations and allows us to relax.
    - Consider methods of relaxation such as meditation, tai chi, yoga, aromatherapy or a massage.
    - Acupuncture can help some people to relax.
    - Make sure that you have some time for yourself to do something you enjoy. There are many forms of entertainment that you may enjoy—for example, go to the cinema or theatre, listen to music, take up a hobby, or go out with friends. Humour can be an effective way of reducing the feelings of stress, so perhaps go and see a funny film or play. When life is difficult time spent with friends and family can be very satisfying.
    - Eat a healthy balanced diet with a lot of fruit and vegetables. Avoid processed foods and foods with high sugar content. This can help mood swings and can help improve your immune system which is often run down during times of stress. Avoid comfort eating if possible—it may make you feel good for a few minutes but then you often feel guilty, increasing your stress levels (see Chapter 20 on how to control comfort eating).
    - Avoid nicotine, caffeine, alcohol, and other stimulants.
    - Try to get enough sleep.
    - Drink plenty of water. If you are mildly dehydrated you can feel lethargic and are unlikely to cope well with pressures.
- Share your concerns
    - Talk to a trusted friend or relative about your worries. They may be able help you to put the stressful events into perspective and even reach a solution.

If you remain extremely stressed or anxious, then do consider going to your doctor and ask to see a counsellor.

8

Treatment of irregular or absent menstrual periods

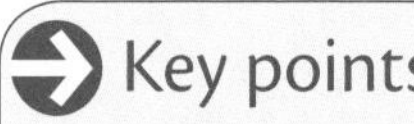

- Over two-thirds of women with PCOS have irregular or absent periods.
- Weight loss if you are overweight may improve the regularity of your periods.
- If you are not trying to become pregnant then the combined contraceptive pill may be prescribed to induce a regular bleed and provide you with contraception. If the contraceptive pill is not appropriate then there are other hormonal treatments your doctor may prescribe to regulate your periods.

Irregular or absent periods is the most common symptom of PCOS, affecting over two-thirds of women. A menstrual period is the result of shedding of the lining of the womb. The womb lining grows in response to oestrogen secretion by the ovaries in preparation for implantation of a fertilized egg. Following ovulation (release of the egg), if the egg is not fertilized then the womb lining is shed. The production of the hormone progesterone following ovulation is essential for the normal shedding of the womb lining. In women with PCOS and infrequent periods, ovulation occurs erratically or not at all. As a result, progesterone is not produced and the womb lining is not shed every month. Periods in many women with PCOS may therefore occur infrequently, known as oligomenorrhoea, and when they do occur they are often painful, heavy, and prolonged.

Some women have *amenorrhoea* which means periods more than 6 months apart. Women with very infrequent periods may develop spotting or bleeding in between periods as the lining of the womb begins to break down. Excessive growth of the lining of the womb may occur in women with less than four periods a year, and over years this can increase the risk of endometrial (womb) cancer. This risk is thought to be present if you are overweight. This is because there is stimulation of growth of the lining of the womb by high blood oestrogen levels as extra oestrogen is made in the fat tissue. For this reason it is important that the womb lining is shed on a regular basis in overweight women with PCOS. However, it is also important to remember that endometrial cancer is a rare complication of PCOS.

If you are currently not trying to become pregnant then treatments to restart ovulation are not necessary as drugs that stimulate ovulation have other side effects and require close monitoring, making their long-term use inappropriate.

What you can do

Excess weight can exacerbate period problems as extra oestrogen made in fat tissues can interfere with ovulation. In addition, the more overweight you are, the more insulin resistant you become, which results in higher testosterone or male hormone levels. Studies have consistently shown that by losing only 5 per cent of your body weight you can improve the frequency of your menstrual cycle and reduce the heaviness of menstrual flow.

What your doctor can do

If you are slim and infrequent periods do not bother you, then you may not need any treatment. However, although you are unlikely to be ovulating regularly you will still need some form of contraception if you are sexually active as you may ovulate occasionally. However, if you are overweight, then you should really aim to have at least 4–6 periods a year to minimize the risk of thickening of the womb lining (Table 8.1). If you are unable, or reluctant, to take any of the treatments available, then your doctor may decide to monitor your womb lining thickness by ultrasound every few years to ensure that it does not grow too thick.

Natural treatments for irregular or absent periods

Vitex agnus-castus, commonly known as Vitex but also called chasteberry, may play a role in treating irregular or absent periods and even premenstrual syndrome. It may reduce breast tenderness, fluid retention, and mood swings premenstrually. The herb is thought to reduce prolactin production by the pituitary gland. Elevated levels of prolactin are found in a number of women with PCOS, and high levels of the hormone prolactin are associated with lack

Table 8.1 The medical treatment of irregular periods

	Side effects	**Notes**
Combined contraceptive pill	◆ Breast tenderness ◆ Nausea ◆ Reduced sex drive ◆ High blood pressure ◆ If you are overweight the contraceptive pill may increase your insulin levels, which may in turn make weight loss more difficult or even cause weight gain. We therefore try to avoid the pill in women who are very overweight ◆ Risk of blood clots, or venous thrombosis, is increased 2- to 3-fold by taking the combined contraceptive pill but remains low in otherwise healthy women at approximately 15–25/100 000 women/year. The risk increases with increasing age, if there is a family history of blood clots, and if you are overweight	◆ Most suitable for slim women. It will also provide you with contraception and may help other symptoms such as greasy skin or acne ◆ Taking the combined contraceptive pill does not affect your fertility. However, it may mask symptoms of PCOS by reducing testosterone levels and its effects on the body. Therefore symptoms, including irregular periods, may become apparent after stopping the pill

(continued)

Table 8.1 The medical treatment of irregular periods *(continued)*

	Side effects	Notes
	◆ Do not use if: • you have previously had a blood clot • you are over the age of 35 years and are a smoker or are overweight • you have high blood pressure or migraines	
Cyclical progestogens, e.g. Provera, Duphaston	◆ Breast tenderness ◆ Bloating ◆ Nausea ◆ Mood swings ◆ Weight gain	◆ Progesterone is the main hormone of the second half of the menstrual cycle. It prepares the womb lining for implantation of the embryo and, if pregnancy does not occur, the falling levels of progesterone result in a period. Progestogens are progesterone-like hormones which are taken for 10–12 days every 1–3 months, the exact type and timing depending upon the woman's individual cycle problem. A menstrual bleed usually follows each course
Cerazette	◆ Nausea ◆ Headache ◆ Breast tenderness	◆ Progesterone-only or 'minipill' may be prescribed if you are unable to take the combined contraceptive pill. Provides you with contraception and may help with period pain ◆ Following a few months of use your periods often become lighter and may stop altogether. However, the womb lining is thinned out so the risk of endometrial cancer is diminished

	◆ Menstrual irregularities ◆ Greasy skin, spots ◆ Weight gain ◆ However, it is less likely to cause side effects compared with other progesterone-only pills. We tend to avoid other 'minipills' in women with PCOS as they have testosterone-like properties and are thus more likely to exacerbate the other symptoms of PCOS	
Metformin	◆ Gastrointestinal—nausea, bloating, diarrhoea and vomiting	◆ Helps to counteract insulin resistance. It is therefore only of use in women who are insulin resistant. Most overweight women with PCOS are insulin resistant but only 30 per cent of slim women have problems with insulin resistance. Research studies have consistently shown that women with PCOS who took metformin were more likely to ovulate and have regular periods than those who did not take it. In some women, normal menstrual cycles may be achieved within 3 months of starting treatment ◆ Please note that by increasing your ovulation, metformin may also enhance your fertility so you do need to use contraception if you do not want to become pregnant ◆ Please see Chapter 6 for more information on metformin

(continued)

Table 8.1 The medical treatment of irregular periods *(continued)*

	Side effects	Notes
Mirena coil	◆ Abdominal pain, especially if you have never had children ◆ Irregular periods initially ◆ The amount of progesterone released is very small so it is far less likely to cause progesterone-associated side effects compared with tablets: • Mood swings • Breast tenderness • Weight gain • Greasy, spotty skin	◆ This is a coil which releases a small amount of progesterone into the womb. The progesterone prevents thickening of the lining of the womb and thus protects from endometrial cancer ◆ Following a few months of use your periods often become lighter and may stop altogether

of periods. Vitex is also known to increase ovarian progesterone production, restoring the balance between oestrogen and progesterone necessary for a normal period. You will need to use Vitex for at least 6 months for the herb's benefits to become apparent. You should not take it if you are taking the contraceptive pill or fertility drugs as it interferes with hormone production and so may affect the efficacy of the treatments.

Dong quai (*Angelica sinensis*) has also been used to restore a normal menstrual cycle and help premenstrual symptoms. Its mechanism of action is not clear.

Licorice root has been shown to reduce testosterone and improve menstruation in two small trials in women with PCOS.

White peony may increase progesterone levels and reduce testosterone levels, thus helping to restore the hormonal imbalance.

We do not recommend that you try and self-prescribe. Since PCOS affects different women differently, the treatments for it in turn should be individualized to you. You should therefore consult a reputable medical herbalist who can assess you, prescribe the appropriate treatment for you, and then monitor you. Additionally, herbal treatments may be associated with side effects which should be explained to you. Some herbs should not be used if you are pregnant or are breastfeeding, and others should not be used if you have other medical conditions or are on certain medication. Your herbalist should discuss all this with you so that you make an informed choice. Finally, your herbalist can also advise you where to buy the supplements as there is a wide variation in the quality of herbs sold at health shops.

9

Treatment of subfertility

Key points

- Infertility affects 10–15% of all couples. Women with PCOS may have problems conceiving if they have irregular periods, indicating that they are not ovulating regularly.
- A healthy balanced diet will optimize your chances of conception. Losing a little weight if you are overweight will also enhance your fertility.
- If your periods remain irregular then your doctor may refer you to a fertility clinic for further investigation and treatment. Treatments are often very successful, but tend to be less effective in women who are very overweight.

Infertility affects 10–15 per cent of all couples. About a third of women who are finding it difficult to become pregnant have problems ovulating, and PCOS is found in approximately 75 per cent of women who are not ovulating. However, please note that many women with PCOS do conceive naturally. If you are finding it difficult to become pregnant then this does not mean you will never be able to have a baby as there are several very effective treatments available. We prefer to use the term subfertility, implying *difficulty* becoming pregnant rather than infertility or *inability* to conceive.

> My husband and I have been trying to conceive for 2 years. I feel so frustrated and have become very tearful, especially when I found out my younger cousin had fallen pregnant.

The reason for infrequent or lack of ovulation is the hormonal imbalance present in women with PCOS, particularly the high insulin and testosterone levels, resulting in failure of the ovarian follicles to mature and release an egg each month. The ovaries can be stimulated to produce eggs again and the treatments have a high chance of success.

What you can do

Sexual intercourse

To give yourselves the best chance of success, you should try to make love every 2–3 days throughout the month. In a normal cycle you tend to ovulate about 14 days before a period. If your periods are irregular, then there is really no point in trying to predict the 'fertile' week as this may be unreliable. Additionally, concentrating your lovemaking on 2–3 days when you think you are most fertile may put a strain on your relationship.

> My partner and I have been trying to conceive for 4 years now. The stress of hospital appointments and investigations are putting a strain on our relationship.

Alcohol and smoking

Both excess alcohol and cigarette smoking have been linked to reduced fertility so you should really stop smoking and ensure that you drink no more than 1–2 units of alcohol a day.

Weight and diet

Women who are significantly overweight can take longer to conceive than women whose weight is in the normal range. If you are overweight and you have irregular or absent periods, losing weight reduces your testosterone and insulin levels, improving your ovulation rate and increasing your chances of becoming pregnant. Even a small reduction in weight may have a beneficial impact on your fertility. Additionally, all treatments to induce ovulation are less successful in women who are very overweight.

Similarly, if you are underweight you may find that if your weight increases up to the normal range for your height your ovaries will start working again and so improve your chances of getting pregnant.

Following a healthy, balanced, and varied diet will ensure you have adequate stores of nutrients to meet your baby's needs during pregnancy. Try to ensure that both you and your partner eat a diet with sufficient amounts of the nutrients listed in Table 9.1 which are thought to enhance fertility. You should also take a folic acid supplement to minimize the risk of neural tube defects in your

Table 9.1 Essential nutrients to optimize conception

Nutrient	Found in
Folic acid	Leafy vegetables (e.g. spinach), oranges
Zinc	Wholegrain cereals, pulses, egg, meat, seafood
Magnesium	Leafy vegetables, wholegrain cereals, dried fruit
Iron	Meat, fish, poultry, seeds, leafy vegetables
Essential fatty acids	Oily fish, flax seed, leafy vegetables
Selenium	Tuna, wholegrain cereals
Vitamin E	Broccoli, leafy vegetables, nuts, wholegrain cereals

baby. You should not need other vitamin or mineral supplements. However, if you want to take a supplement, choose a multivitamin or mineral supplement that is specifically for women seeking pregnancy as this is more likely to provide nutrients in balanced amounts, not high doses that may be dangerous to your baby's health. You should avoid supplements containing vitamin A as this has been linked with birth defects. We would not recommend taking any herbal supplements if you are trying to conceive unless you are under the supervision of a qualified and reputable medical herbalist.

What your doctor can do

If you have regular periods and are under the age of 35 years, then you should see your doctor if you have been unable to conceive following a year of regular unprotected intercourse. However, if you have irregular periods or are over the age of 35 years and have not been able to get pregnant after 6 months of regular lovemaking, then you should see your doctor. Although not ovulating is likely to be the cause of your subfertility, it is important to check for other possible causes in yourself or your partner before starting any treatment. Your doctor will probably ask for a semen sample from your partner to check his sperm count and the health of his sperm, and will also check your hormones. If you are having periods, your doctor will probably assess whether or not you are ovulating by measuring blood progesterone levels 7 days after presumed ovulation. Progesterone is produced by the empty follicle following normal ovulation.

He/she will probably then refer you to a specialist clinic for further investigations as necessary and for treatment. The most common tests are shown in Table 9.2. Please note that treatments for subfertility are less likely to be effective if you are very overweight, and so most hospitals restrict treatments until you have lost some weight (Table 9.3).

Table 9.2 Investigation of subfertility

Test	Notes
Semen analysis	A normal semen analysis will show more than 20 million sperm/ml of which >60% will be motile and <40% will be abnormal
Day 21 progesterone	This is measured to assess ovulation. A level of over 10 confirms ovulation
FSH, LH, prolactin, testosterone	FSH is often used as a gauge of ovarian reserve. Its levels are usually normal in women with PCOS but the level rises in women going through an early menopause. An LH that is higher than FSH or a high testosterone level are indicators of PCOS. Increased prolactin levels can interfere with ovulation and are found in about 30% of women with PCOS
Thyroid function tests	If you have an untreated over- or underactive thyroid gland this can affect your fertility
Laparoscopy	This is done under a general anaesthetic to look at the ovaries, Fallopian tubes, and uterus. The doctor will insert a telescope through a small incision inside the belly button or just below it. A laparoscopy is performed to exclude conditions such as endometriosis and adhesions which can cause blocked tubes. It is likely to be performed as a day case

Patients' perspectives

Lisa, aged 35, was diagnosed with PCOS when she went to her GP complaining that she had not had a period for 9 months. This was making her increasingly depressed as she had been trying for a baby for a year. When Lisa came to clinic she weighed 132 kg (20 stone 12 lb). It was recommended that she tried to lose weight by following the principles of the low-GI diet and increasing her physical activity. She was also prescribed metformin and had a period 6 weeks later! By 4 months she had lost 10 kg (24 lb) in weight, her periods were regular, and her mood was a lot better. By 12 months Lisa had lost 21 kg (4 stone) and became pregnant. She gave birth to her baby daughter earlier this year.

Angela, aged 36, was increasingly worried. She had been trying to conceive for 18 months. She became pregnant once but unfortunately had a miscarriage. She was slim but did have irregular periods as a teenager. The diagnosis of PCOS was made when she was investigated for subfertility. She then read about the low-GI principles and introduced it to her diet. In clinic she was prescribed metformin and became pregnant 3 months later. She now has a beautiful baby boy.

Problems during pregnancy

It is important to remember that once you become pregnant you will probably have a normal and uncomplicated pregnancy. However, there are a couple of problems that occasionally develop if you have PCOS.

It is estimated that in the general population one pregnancy in five ends in a miscarriage, mostly in the first 12 weeks of pregnancy. If you have PCOS, the risk may be increased. The most common cause for a miscarriage is an abnormal embryo. In PCOS, having high insulin or LH levels may increase the risk of miscarriage as the hormonal imbalance results in poorer egg quality. The high hormonal levels may also reduce progesterone production which is essential for preparation of the womb lining in order to provide a place for your embryo to attach. It is therefore important that you try and keep your insulin levels down, as discussed in Chapter 6. Although treatment remains unlicensed, there is some evidence that in insulin-resistant pregnant women with PCOS continuing metformin until the 12th week of pregnancy may reduce the risk of miscarriage by reducing insulin and LH levels. Currently there is no evidence to suggest that the use of metformin during pregnancy increases abnormalities in the baby. If you have been unfortunate enough to have two or more miscarriages, then you will probably need investigating for other causes of recurrent miscarriages. Miscarriages can be very traumatic and distressing, and you must make sure that you ask for the support you need from friends, family and trained counsellors.

If you have PCOS, particularly if you are overweight, then you are at increased risk of developing gestational diabetes (diabetes in pregnancy). You should therefore ensure that you are screened for this, usually by 24 weeks of pregnancy and then again later in pregnancy. This will involve two blood sugar tests—one fasting and the other 2 hours after a meal or a glucose drink (glucose tolerance test). If you do develop diabetes in pregnancy, then this is often managed by controlling your diet. However, if this does not keep your blood sugars under control, then you may need insulin for the remaining duration of the pregnancy as high blood sugar levels are passed through the placenta to the developing baby. Having high blood sugar can cause the baby to grow larger, which can make delivery difficult and potentially cause injuries to both

Table 9.3 Fertility treatments in PCOS

	Side effects	Notes
Metformin	◆ Gastrointestinal—nausea, bloating, diarrhoea and vomiting	◆ We would suggest a 6 month trial of metformin if you are insulin resistant. Trials have shown it to be effective in many insulin-resistant women with PCOS with no risk of complications such as multiple pregnancy or ovarian hyperstimulation. It may also reduce the risk of miscarriage if continued up until 13 weeks of pregnancy ◆ If ovulation does not resume within 6 months or you do not become pregnant, then other fertility drugs may be added ◆ Metformin may improve your response to other fertility treatments such as clomiphene
Clomiphene	◆ Hot flushes, mood swings, depression, headaches, pelvic pain ◆ Multiple pregnancy in up to 10% ◆ 1% risk of ovarian hyperstimulation (see below) ◆ Ideally ovarian follicle growth should be monitored by regular ultrasound to minimize the risk of multiple pregnancies and ovarian hyperstimulation ◆ It is recommended that you have a maximum of 12 cycles of clomiphene as use beyond this may be associated with an increased risk of ovarian cancer	◆ Clomiphene stimulates the body's own supply of FSH from the pituitary gland. It is given in tablet form and is usually prescribed for 5 days shortly after the start of a period ◆ In women with PCOS, 70% will ovulate using clomiphene and in those who ovulate, 50% will conceive within 6 months

Ovarian diathermy	• Involves a general anaesthetic • Abdominal pain and pain below the shoulder blades • Nausea • Vaginal bleeding • Rarely—adhesion formation or ovarian failure if there is a complication	• This is a procedure performed by laparoscopic, or 'keyhole', surgery in which several tiny holes are burnt on the surfaces of the ovaries with a laser or using an electric current. We do not know why, but following this the hormonal imbalance is often corrected and ovulation restored, at least temporarily. It has an ovulation rate of >80% and a pregnancy rate of >50%, particularly in slim women with PCOS • Following ovarian diathermy, your response to clomiphene or metformin may improve
Gonadotrophins	• Abdominal distension, bloating sensation, mood swings, fatigue. • Risk of multiple pregnancy (20%) so you will need careful monitoring with ultrasound to ensure only one follicle matures. • Ovarian hyperstimulation syndrome may develop if you are very sensitive to gonadotrophins and produce a large number of follicles. The ovaries become quite enlarged and then leak fluid into the abdominal cavity resulting in a lot of abdominal pain. Women with PCOS are particularly susceptible to this. It can be life threatening and so careful monitoring using blood tests and ultrasound is essential in any woman given gonadotrophins to stimulate ovulation	• Given as a daily injection • Ovulation rates of >90% and pregnancy rates of 70% after six cycles

(continued)

Table 9.3 Fertility treatments in PCOS *(continued)*

	Side effects	Notes
In vitro fertilization (IVF)	◆ This can be physically and emotionally very demanding, and a substantial time commitment is required by both partners ◆ Hot flushes when receiving drugs to switch off your hormones ◆ Hyperstimulation of the ovaries or failure of the ovaries to respond ◆ Pain during egg retrieval ◆ Multiple pregnancy if more than one embryo is inserted in your womb ◆ Expensive if it is not offered on the NHS in your area	◆ You will initially need hormone treatment to switch off your hormones, followed by injections to stimulate egg production in a controlled manner. Eggs that have been stimulated to maturity are collected from the ovaries by needle through the vaginal wall, guided by ultrasound. The eggs are then fertilized in the laboratory by your partner's sperm. After 2 or 3 days the fertilized eggs (embryos) are transferred to the womb ◆ The overall pregnancy rate per treatment cycle is 25% if you are under 38 years of age

mother and baby during birth. There are other risks to the baby's health if the blood sugars are not brought under control such as low blood sugars shortly after delivery. These risks are minimized by keeping your blood sugars under control during pregnancy. If you develop gestational diabetes, this usually goes away after delivery but your risk of developing type 2 diabetes is increased significantly. You should have a glucose tolerance test at around 6 weeks after your baby is born to make sure you do not have type 2 diabetes and, if this is normal, you will need annual blood sugar checks to screen for diabetes.

10

Treatment of excess body hair

Key points

- Up to 28% of all women in the UK suffer from unwanted facial hair. Approximately 70% of women with PCOS develop unwanted hair at some stage of their lives.
- Excess hair growth can be treated successfully using medication. However, hair regrowth usually occurs when treatment is stopped.
- There is no evidence that any form of hair removal will result in more hair growth. Laser hair removal and electrolysis are often effective in producing a long-lasting reduction in hair growth although several sessions will be required.

Hirsutism is the presence of excess facial or body hair in women in a male-pattern distribution. It is a common complaint, with one study showing that up to 28 per cent of all women in the UK suffer from unwanted facial hair. PCOS is the most common cause of hirsutism. Approximately 70 per cent of women with PCOS develop unwanted hair at some stage of their lives. If you spend an hour a week secretly tweezering out unwanted facial hair, it can be particularly distressing and can make you feel very self-conscious. We have fine hair all over our body except on our palms and soles. In some women, hairs in certain parts may grow darker and coarser, and become more obvious. So, typically, dark hairs may grow on the upper lip and chin, around the nipples, on the tops of the shoulders and thighs. Pubic hair growth may extend upward to the middle of the abdomen.

> My facial hair was ruining my life. I wore polo necks, even during summer, to hide my hair as I felt so self-conscious.

Hair growth

In order for you to understand how the different treatments for excess body hair work and why they take time to take effect, it is important for you to know a little about how hair grows. Each hair grows from a funnel in the skin called a hair follicle. Sebaceous (oil) glands are connected to the follicle, and the sebum, or oil, that is secreted serves to condition the hair. We are all born with approximately 5 million hair follicles covering our body. No more follicles develop after birth although the size of the follicles, and thus the nature of the hairs, is influenced by hormones, particularly androgens or male-type sex hormones. There are two types of hair—*vellus* and *terminal*. Vellus hair is the fine short downy hair located on most parts of your body. Terminal hair is coarser, pigmented, and longer, and is located on the scalp, eyebrows, and eyelashes. At puberty, small amounts of androgens produced by the adrenal glands stimulate terminal hair growth under the armpits and in the pubic area. There is a mixture of vellus and terminal hairs on the lower legs and forearms of all women, which is usually determined by your genes and your ethnic origin rather than by hormones. If you have high levels of male hormone in the blood or your skin is more sensitive to testosterone, then you may also develop terminal hairs in a male-type distribution, for example on the chin, upper lip, chest, or inner thighs (Fig. 10.1). This is hirsutism and occurs when vellus hairs are changed to terminal hairs as a result of the skin's excess sensitivity to testosterone. Only androgen-dependent hair growth, or hirsutism, will respond to hormonal treatment. The change of vellus hair to terminal hair is usually permanent, and so it is important to treat hirsutism as early as possible to prevent further terminal hairs from growing. Androgens also increase sebum, or oil production, resulting in greasy skin, spots, and acne.

Every hair follicle undergoes three phases of a growth cycle.

- The *anagen* phase is the growth stage. Hair length is determined by the length of anagen and varies in different areas of the body. Each body hair grows for about 3 months while scalp hair grows for up to 3 years.
- This is followed by the *catagen*, or resting, phase.
- Finally, the hair is shed in the *telegen* phase. The cells at the base of the hair follicle then begin to divide and form a new hair and the cycle starts again.

So if you pluck a hair, as long as the follicle is not completely destroyed, a new hair will grow in its place. Hair follicles are in different phases of the growth cycle at any one time—about 85 per cent are growing, 1 per cent are

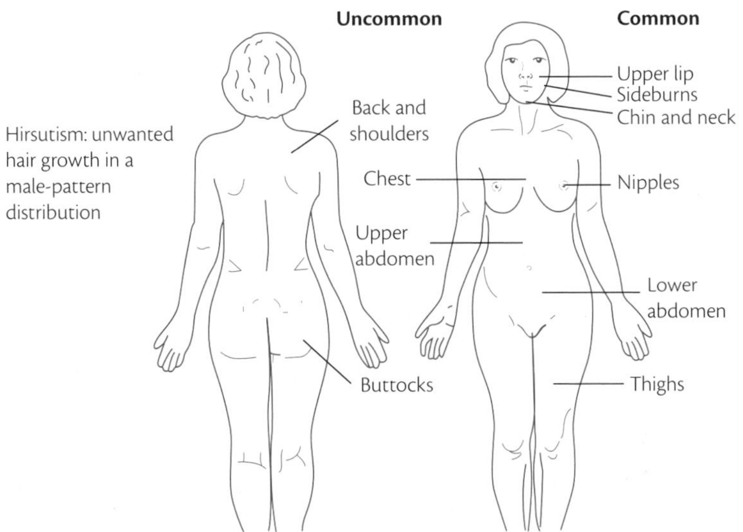

Figure 10.1 Androgen-sensitive sites of hair growth.

resting and 14 per cent are moulting. Some drugs or hormonal conditions may synchronize hair growth. For example, during pregnancy you may notice that your scalp hair appears thicker. This is because more hairs are in the anagen phase than usual and so hair appears thicker. Then, for the first 6 months or so after delivery, hairs tend to shed more than usual as more hairs enter the telegen phase. Electrolysis and laser hair removal only damage follicles when the hairs are in the anagen, or growth, phase, which is why several sessions are required to reduce hair growth permanently in one area.

Why does hirsutism develop in women with PCOS?

The ovaries and adrenal glands (which are small glands lying just above the kidneys) produce some male hormone in all adult women. Women with PCOS often produce a higher than usual amount of testosterone, mainly by the ovaries. Additionally, women with PCOS are often more sensitive to the effects of testosterone than usual, at least partly because of the lower level of sex hormone-binding globulin (SHBG). This is a protein which carries sex hormones in the blood. Androgens and high insulin levels decrease the amount of SHBG. If there is less SHBG, more of the testosterone is 'free' (unbound to protein) and available to act on the hair follicles. Testosterone stimulates the conversion of the fine vellus hairs into coarser and thicker terminal hairs in androgen-sensitive skin. There are other factors affecting a woman's susceptibility to hirsutism. For example, it often runs in the family, and certain races, particularly women of Asian origin, are more susceptible than others. Hirsutism varies in severity from very mild, having to pluck the odd hair, to more severe, spending an hour removing hair daily.

What you can do

If you are overweight, you are likely to be insulin resistant and the high insulin levels will increase male hormone production while reducing SHBG levels. This will tend to stimulate body hair production. Losing weight and increasing your physical activity will reduce your insulin and, subsequently, testosterone levels. This may help control unwanted hair growth and will also help your health in general.

There are a number of physical methods of hair removal, which may be all that you need if your hirsutism is mild. If you have a lot of excess hair, then you may need to consult your doctor to combine physical methods with hormonal therapies. Table 10.1 lists the available options for hair removal. There is no evidence that any form of hair removal will result in more hair growth, although hairs do look coarser if you shave.

Before you go ahead with electrolysis ...

- Do choose a reputable therapist as if it is performed incorrectly scarring can occur. Choose a therapist registered with the British Institute and Association of Electrolysis or go by word of mouth. All premises at which electrolysis is carried out should be registered with the local authority which will enforce rigid standards of hygiene and sterility.

- Avoid clinics which do not offer a free consultation. A professional clinic will take the time to determine the treatment most suited to your individual needs and to make sure you know all about what it will involve before the course begins.

- Do ask about costs and how many treatments you can expect to need. Expect to go every 1–2 weeks initially. The frequency and the time spent on each session will diminish as the hairs respond to treatment. The reason for needing several sessions is that only hairs in the 'growth' phase will respond to treatment. Since hair grows in cycles, not all of the hairs are in the growth phase at any given time. The length of the treatment course will depend on the amount of hair present. If you have a lot of hair, do see

Table 10.1 Methods of hair removal

	Best for	Advantages	Disadvantages
Bleaching	Face, especially upper lip	◆ Easy, cheap, painless	◆ Skin irritation
Shaving	Legs and underarms	◆ Easy, quick, cheap, painless	◆ Short-lasting effects and can cause stubble so you may have to shave daily ◆ Can cause skin irritation, cuts, and ingrowing hairs
Plucking	Odd stray hair on face or chest	◆ Easy, cheap	◆ Only suitable for a few stray hairs otherwise time consuming and painful ◆ Can result in ingrowing hairs and infection, which can cause spots and scarring
Depilatory creams	Underarms, legs Face—use a face-specific cream to avoid irritation Inexpensive	◆ Easy, quick ◆ Smooth finish for days	◆ Skin rash or irritation ◆ Messy
Waxing or sugaring Hot wax or sugary paste is applied to the skin which is then removed by a strip of cloth, taking hairs with it	Legs, underarms, bikini line, face	◆ Longer-lasting results (up to 6 weeks) ◆ Smooth finish	◆ Painful. Can result in ingrowing hairs and infection, which can cause spots ◆ Skin irritation ◆ Have to leave hair to grow long enough before waxing/sugaring

(continued)

Table 10.1 Methods of hair removal *(continued)*

	Best for	Advantages	Disadvantages
Epilators An electric device with rows of tweezers on a rotating head, used like an electric shaver but pulls hairs out at the root	Legs, arms	◆ Longer-lasting results ◆ Smooth finish	◆ Painful ◆ Can result in ingrowing hairs and infection which can cause spots and scarring, skin irritation ◆ Have to leave hair to grow long enough for tweezers to grasp
Electrolysis A small electric current is applied to each hair follicle using a needle or probe, destroying the hair root.	Face, bikini line	◆ May experience long-lasting or permanent hair removal ◆ Treatment is not restricted to certain hair and skin colours	◆ Expensive ◆ Painful ◆ Time consuming—will need several sessions ◆ Only really suitable to treat small areas ◆ Can cause scarring if not performed by a trained and reputable therapist ◆ Please note that home electrolysis kits are not usually effective as the current used is too low to destroy the hair root

Laser Light at a specified wavelength is applied to the hair follicle which is then absorbed by the hair pigment. The heat energy from the laser light destroys the follicle. Is most effective if you are fair skinned with dark hair. There are different lasers around, emitting light of different wavelengths. The most commonly used are Nd:YAG, ruby, and alexandrite lasers	Face, legs, bikini line, arms, underarms	◆ May experience long-lasting hair removal ◆ May be used to treat large areas of the body ◆ Less painful than electrolysis	◆ Grey or blonde hair is unlikely to respond. The laser energy may also destroy pigment (melanin) in the skin around the hair, so you could end up with pale skin patches. This is most likely if you have dark skin. Dark skin patches, or hyperpigmentation, may also occur. Expensive, several sessions required as laser only destroys hairs that are currently in the growth cycle ◆ There must be hair in the follicle in order for it to be effective, so avoid plucking or waxing prior to treatment—however, you can shave unwanted hair ◆ May experience redness or stinging but this usually settles within 1–2 days ◆ Avoid the sun for at least 3–4 weeks before the procedure. ◆ Avoid if you have had isotretinoin (Roaccutane) to treat acne over the preceding 6 months
Intense pulsed light (IPL) Filtered light is applied to the skin which is then absorbed by the pigment in the hair follicle, destroying it			

your doctor. He/she may refer you to a dermatologist (skin specialist) or endocrinologist (hormone specialist) who can assess whether you need medical treatment. It may be more cost-effective to delay electrolysis until after you have had 12 months of medical treatment.

- Unfortunately electrolysis is not available on the NHS.

Before you go ahead with laser or IPL therapy ...

- Do choose a reputable therapist as if it is performed incorrectly burning and scarring can occur. Always choose a clinic which is registered with the Healthcare Commission. This ensures that the clinic is inspected regularly and conforms to a minimum standard of safety and care. Never go to an unregistered clinic.

- Avoid clinics which do not offer a free consultation and a test patch to test for skin reactions and effectiveness before you commit yourself financially. A professional clinic will take the time to determine the treatment most suited to your individual needs and to make sure you know all about what it will involve before the course begins.

- Make sure you understand how you will be charged for the treatment. A good clinic will allow you the option to pay as you go instead of in advance.

- The number of treatment sessions needed is usually between 6 and 12, depending on the amount of hair present. After completing your treatment you can hope for up to 70 per cent reduction in hair growth rather than permanent hair removal, but the hairs that grow back tend to be finer. If you have a lot of hair, do see your doctor. He/she may refer you to a dermatologist (skin specialist) or endocrinologist (hormone specialist) who can assess whether you need medical treatment. It may be more cost-effective to delay laser or intensive pulse light (IPL) hair removal until after you have had 12 months of medical treatment.

- Unfortunately laser and IPL are not available on the NHS in all counties although health authorities are increasingly making it available to women with PCOS, so do ask your doctor who can advise you about availability in your area.

When to go to your doctor

Living with hirsutism can be distressing. You may feel unfeminine and self-conscious about your excessive hair growth. Even though you may be embarrassed, it is very important that you talk to your doctor to discuss the treatments available. Ask if you could see a female doctor at the surgery if that would make you feel more comfortable. It is also important for you to understand that PCOS and hirsutism are very common problems experienced by many women.

I am too embarrassed to go to my doctor about my excess hair growth and it is making my life a misery.

- If there is a sudden increase in your hair growth or you develop a deepening of your voice then you must see your doctor. You will probably need to be investigated to make sure there is nothing else causing your symptoms.
- If you have other symptoms from PCOS then you should see your doctor so that you can be assessed and the most appropriate management plan can be agreed.
- If you are having to spend a lot of money on electrolysis or laser treatment, are depressed and worried by your appearance, or are finding it difficult to keep your symptoms under control, then you should see your doctor who will be able to discuss the various medical treatments with you.

What your doctor can do

He/she may refer you to an endocrinologist (hormone specialist) for further tests and treatment. If you have not yet been diagnosed with PCOS your doctor or the endocrinologist may want to arrange blood tests and an ultrasound scan to confirm the diagnosis. If the endocrinologist is concerned that your unwanted hair may be caused by another condition, then he/she will arrange the relevant tests before starting treatment.

There are various treatment options available, but please remember that risks of treatment should be weighed against any likely benefit (Table 10.2). Your endocrinologist will take a detailed medical history and examine you to assess which of the treatments are most suitable for you. He/she is also in the best position to monitor you as necessary. Medications which block the effects of male hormones, or androgens, are most commonly used to reduce hirsutism. The treatments are effective in a large number of women but do take time to work, and therefore you may not notice much of an effect for the first 6 months. Then the hairs will grow more slowly and finer and you may notice that you are having to remove your hair less often. If one treatment does not work, it may be worth trying another. Unfortunately the moment the drug is stopped hair tends to grow back. Before stopping drug treatment, therefore, it is advisable that you consider a course of laser, IPL, or electrolysis to minimize hair regrowth. Please note that you must not take male hormone blockers when pregnant or trying for a baby as they can harm the foetus. You must therefore use contraception if you are sexually active and on anti-androgens or male hormone blockers. Finally, although we do not know of any long-term ill effects from the treatments, none is officially licensed for the treatment of hirsutism or PCOS.

Please note that any of the treatments for PCOS must be instigated by a doctor who can help you decide which treatment is best for you, make sure that you have no medical condition precluding you from taking the drug, and ensure that you receive the appropriate monitoring.

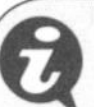

Patients' perspectives

Hannah, aged 19 years, was seen in the PCOS clinic. Her main complaint was excess facial and body hair. She had to shave her face twice a day and still felt self-conscious about her facial stubble. At her first clinic visit she weighed 80 kg (12 stone 8 lb) and did have evidence of excessive hair growth on her face, chest, and lower tummy. The low-GI diet was recommended and metformin prescribed. When she was seen 4 months later she had lost 12 kg (2 stone) but her hair growth was not much better. She was then put on spironolactone in addition to metformin. A year after she first presented to clinic she weighed 57 kg (9 stone) and her hirsutism was a lot better. The hairs on her body were a lot finer and did not need removing and Hannah was now shaving her face only once a week.

Amirah, aged 22 years, complained of excessive facial hair after stopping the contraceptive pill a year earlier. She was spending 15 minutes a day plucking her facial hair. Vaniqa was prescribed, and within 4 months Amirah's facial hair had diminished so much that she only had to pluck the odd hair once every 7–10 days.

Sally, aged 26 years, was diagnosed with PCOS in her late teens when she was being investigated for irregular periods and acne. She was put on Dianette for 5 years. However, since stopping the treatment, she had noticed increasing facial hair which she was plucking twice a week. She opted for six sessions of laser hair removal. A year following the treatment her facial hair had not regrown.

Table 10.2 Treatment of hirsutism

Drug	Efficacy	Side effects	Notes
Combined contraceptive pill **—Dianette** **—Yasmin** Suppress testosterone production by the ovaries and increase SHBG production so there is less free testosterone to act on the skin	◆ Useful for mild hirsutism ◆ May need to add a stronger male hormone blocker if there is an inadequate response	◆ Dianette can enhance weight gain and can cause mood swings. ◆ Breast tenderness ◆ Nausea ◆ Reduced sex drive	◆ Do not use if: • you have previously had a blood clot • you are over the age of 35 years and are a smoker or are overweight • you have high blood pressure or migraines ◆ Yasmin is a relatively new drug so we do not know whether it is as effective as Dianette in treating acne or excess hair growth
Vaniqa Acts by blocking one of the enzymes essential for normal hair growth Effects usually seen within 8–12 weeks of use	◆ New cream licensed only for facial hirsutism ◆ It is effective in reducing hair growth in 70% of women with mild/moderate hirsutism	◆ Acne ◆ An allergic skin rash	◆ Almost invariably a minute amount of the active ingredient will be absorbed into the bloodstream so it should not be used if you are pregnant or trying to become pregnant

(continued)

Table 10.2 Treatment of hirsutism (*continued*)

Drug	Efficacy	Side effects	Notes
Metformin Insulin sensitizer. The fall in insulin levels results in a reduction in ovarian testosterone production and a rise in SHBG so there is less free testosterone to act on the skin	◆ May be effective in mild to moderate hirsutism. ◆ In more severe hirsutism, add-on treatment is often necessary.	◆ Nausea ◆ Bloatedness ◆ Diarrhoea, vomiting	◆ Do not use if you have liver or kidney disease. ◆ Your liver and kidney function will need regular monitoring. ◆ Unlikely to be effective if you are not insulin resistant.
Spironolactone Antiandrogen—blocks the effects of testosterone on the skin. May also reduce testosterone production by the ovaries.	◆ Very effective in 80% of women if used in high doses	◆ It can cause erratic periods, so is often given with a contraceptive pill. ◆ Is a diuretic (increases your urine volume) ◆ It can affect potassium levels in the blood so close monitoring is required.	◆ Do not use if you have high potassium levels or abnormal kidney function ◆ You must use contraception if you are sexually active. ◆ Your potassium and kidney function should be checked regularly.

Cyproterone acetate Anti-androgen—blocks the effects of testosterone on the skin	◆ Very effective in over 80% of women	◆ Tiredness ◆ Weight gain ◆ Mood changes ◆ Reduced sex drive ◆ Absent periods if you are on too high a dose ◆ Rarely—abnormal liver function	◆ Do not use if: • you have had a blood clot in the past • you are overweight • you have liver problems • you suffer or have suffered from depression ◆ Usually taken 10 days a month in combination with a contraceptive pill. You must use contraception if you are sexually active ◆ Liver function must be checked regularly
Flutamide Anti-androgen—blocks the effects of testosterone on the skin	◆ As effective as spironolactone.	◆ Dry skin ◆ Weight gain	◆ Rarely used in the UK as it has been associated with fatal liver disease. If used then your liver function must be monitored regularly ◆ You must use contraception if you are sexually active
Finasteride Blocks the conversion of testosterone to a more active androgen in the skin	◆ Appears to be as effective as spironolactone	◆ Headache ◆ Low mood	◆ You must use contraception if you are sexually active

Natural treatments for hirsutism

A healthy diet, increasing physical activity, and stress management will significantly improve your insulin sensitivity, resulting in a fall in insulin levels and a corresponding fall in testosterone production by the ovaries. In the long term this should reduce excess body hair growth.

There is some anecdotal evidence that some herbs may help reduce excess hair growth. However, most of these have not been assessed by proper scientific studies so their efficacy is really unknown.

- **Black cohosh** is thought to reduce LH, thereby reducing ovarian androgen production.
- **Saw palmetto** is thought to work by reducing testosterone action.
- **Green tea** may also reduce the effects of testosterone on the body.
- **White peony** may reduce testosterone levels.

Even though these products are considered 'natural', if they are potent enough to cause a hormonal change in the body, then they are potent enough to cause side effects in some women and may react with any medication you may be taking. You really should see a reputable herbalist or clinical nutritionist who can assess you, discuss the most suitable treatments for you, prescribe the appropriate doses, and monitor you. He/she can also advise you where to buy the supplements as unfortunately there is a wide variation in the quality of over-the-counter nutritional and herbal supplements.

Summary

Hirsutism or excess body hair is a common problem in women, particularly if you have PCOS. It can be treated successfully using anti-androgens or male hormone blockers, although it may take several months to see an effect. Treatment is most effective the earlier it is started. Metformin may also help to treat hirsutism although it does not appear to be as effective as anti-androgens. Vaniqa is a new topical cream increasingly being used to treat facial hirsutism with good effect. A combination of treatments may produce the best results. All drug treatments must be instigated and prescribed by a doctor, and anti-androgens and Vaniqa must not be used without contraception if you are sexually active. Medical treatment should be combined with mechanical methods of hair removal, none of which increase hair growth. The method of hair removal is therefore dependent on personal preference. Electrolysis, laser therapy, or IPL therapy may produce long-lasting hair removal if they are used after a course of medical treatment.

11

Treatment of hair loss

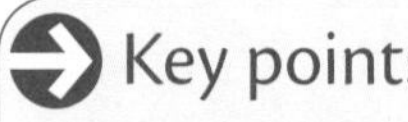

Key points

- Approximately 10 per cent of women with PCOS suffer from hair thinning but fortunately this rarely progresses to baldness.
- A well-balanced nutritious diet is important for healthy hair.
- Although there is no cure for hair loss there are medical treatments available which reduce hair loss and encourage hair regrowth. However, hair thinning tends to recur when treatment is stopped.

Hair loss is a big worry to many people. It is relatively common in women, with a recent survey suggesting that 1.6 million British women have problems with hair loss. Another survey revealed that significant hair loss in women can be so devastating that it can cause depression and relationship break-ups. We all lose about 100 hairs a day, particularly during shampooing and brushing our hair. If you have noticed a persistently larger number of hairs than usual in the plughole after showering, then perhaps you should see your doctor. There are several common treatable conditions which may result in temporary hair loss (Table 11.1). If these conditions are excluded and hair thinning is related to PCOS, then your doctor may refer you to a dermatologist (skin specialist) or endocrinologist (hormone specialist). Approximately 1 in 10 women with PCOS suffer from *androgenic alopecia* or 'male-pattern' hair loss and, if severe, this can cause a great deal of psychological suffering. Androgenic alopecia is diagnosed if hair is thinning from the temples and crown.

> I have noticed that I have been losing a lot of hair. When I run my hands through my hair I get a clump of hairs with it. I used to have very thick hair but my hair is gradually getting thinner.

Table 11.1 Causes of temporary hair loss

Severe stress
Poor diet—especially protein, iron, vitamin B and zinc deficiencies
Illnesses, e.g. febrile illness, surgery, rapid weight changes
Hormonal abnormalities—thyroid disease
Anaemia
Medications, e.g. antithyroid pills, blood thinners, some antidepressants
Postnatally

Hair growth

We each have about 100 000 hairs on our scalp. Remember, there are three phases in the hair growth cycle. The growth or anagen phase of scalp hair lasts between 2 and 6 years (anagen phase). This is followed by the catagen, or resting, phase. Finally, the hair falls out in the telegen phase, a new hair grows, and the cycle starts again (Fig. 11.1). On a healthy head, about 90 per cent of hairs are in the growth, or anagen, phase, 1 per cent are in the resting phase, and the other 9 per cent are in the telegen, or moulting, phase. Excessive hair loss usually occurs if the anagen phase is shortened and the telegen phase is lengthened. This can eventually lead to the hair follicles shutting down completely. Hair loss is often age related. It is normal to lose hair from our early thirties, and by the age of 50 over half of all women have generalized thinning of their hair.

Hair growth is controlled by our genes and hormones. For example, female hormones, or oestrogens, tend to make hair grow longer and thicker, as happens in pregnancy. After the menopause, hair thinning becomes more evident, partly as a result of declining oestrogen levels. You are more likely to suffer from thinning hair if either your parents or grandparents suffered from hair loss. Whereas testosterone stimulates hair growth on the face, chest, and abdomen, it can cause hair thinning on the scalp. The skin of the scalp converts testosterone to another substance called dihydrotestosterone (DHT). Hair follicles on the top of the head and the temples are especially sensitive to DHT. It makes them shrink, and hairs grow progressively shorter and thinner, resulting in male-pattern hair thinning. Hair starts thinning from the sides of the forehead and the crown. Male-pattern hair thinning (androgenic alopecia) can affect women too, but fortunately this rarely progresses to total or near baldness.

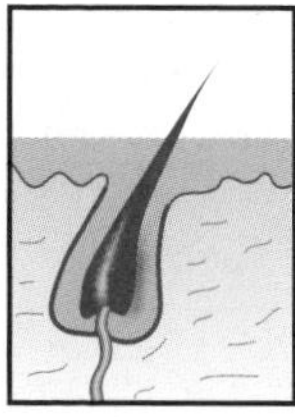

Anagen phase

Growth phase (2–6 years)

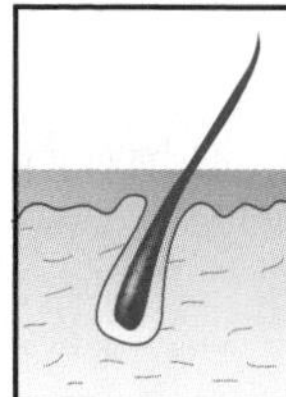

Catagen phase

Resting phase (2 weeks)
Hair stops growing

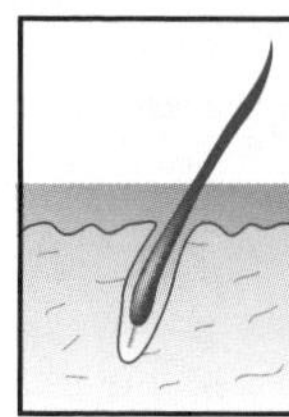

Telegen phase

Hair is shed during this phase
and new hair grows in its place
Lasts 10–16 weeks

Figure 11.1 The hair growth cycle.

Male-pattern hair thinning may occur in women with PCOS in response to higher levels of testosterone and also increased sensitivity of the hair follicles to testosterone. However, please do not worry—it is unlikely that you will become completely bald.

What you can do

- Look after your hair and scalp After washing don't rub your hair vigorously or use a hot hairdryer. Instead, pat it dry with a soft towel or use a low setting on the dryer or, even better, let it dry naturally. Use a brush with soft bristles. Undo any tangles with your fingers, rather than pulling with a comb. Do not brush your hair when wet.

- Wash your hair once or twice a week with a mild shampoo; dirty hair lies flatter and looks more sparse. Change your shampoo and conditioner from time to time to avoid build-up.

- Go to the very best hair stylist for advice on your hair. Be ready to change the colour and style you've always worn. Flat close-to-the-head styles can make hair look thinner. Short, bouncy, curly, or wavy styles can add the illusion of fullness.

Myths about hair loss

Myth: Frequent shampooing may increase hair loss.

Fact: shampooing simply gets rid of the hairs that have already fallen out, giving the appearance of excess shedding in the shower.

Myth: Hats and wigs cause hair loss.

Fact: wigs and hats will only damage hair if they are too tight.

Myth: Brushing your hair 100 strokes a day will create healthier hair.

Fact: vigorous brushing is more likely to injure the hairs and make the problem worse.

Myth: Permanent hair loss is caused by perms, colours, and other cosmetic treatments.

Fact: hair dyes, perms and hairsprays do not affect thinning hair. In fact perms and hairsprays can help to disguise the problem. However, if the treatments are too strong, they may cause the hair to break off near the scalp.

Myth: Shaving your hair will make it grow back thicker.

Fact: hair grows at an average rate of half an inch per month. Cutting hair has absolutely no effect on each hair's thickness or the number of hairs that will sprout from the follicles.

Myth: Certain shampoos and conditioners can cause the hair to grow thicker and faster.

Fact: certain conditioners temporarily fill in defects on the surface of the hair shaft, making it appear smoother and thicker.

Myth: Stress causes permanent hair loss.

Fact: severe stress can affect hair growth but its effect is temporary.

Myth: Hair loss does not occur in the late teens or early twenties.

Fact: hair loss can occur as early as in the mid teens, although fortunately this is rare.

Myth: There is a cure for androgenic alopecia.

Fact: there are no cures for hair loss. Many people waste time and money on treatments advertised on the Internet which claim to make hair regrow, or to stop further hair loss. Most have not been assessed by proper research studies and sadly the majority do not work.

Natural treatments for hair loss in PCOS

Healthy hair requires good nutrition with enough iron, vitamins, especially vitamins B and C, zinc, and essential fatty acids (Table 11.2). A recent survey showed that a significant number of women under the age of 55 do not take the recommended levels of several minerals and nutrients in their diets. Do try to ensure you are taking enough protein in your diet, at least two portions of oily fish a week, and enough of the nutrients listed in Table 11.2.

If you are worried that your diet may be deficient, then you could take a supplement. You may need a supplement, for example, if you are on a low-carbohydrate diet and not eating enough fruit or vegetables. However, it is easy to overdose oneself with over-the-counter vitamins which can be harmful, for example if you take too much iron or vitamin A. It is therefore always best to obtain the bulk of your vitamin and mineral requirements from your diet. Taking dietary supplements has not been shown to reduce hair loss unless your diet is very deficient.

Table 11.2 Nutrients necessary for healthy hair

Nutrient	Found in
Biotin	Milk, liver, oats, brown rice, peas, lentils, sunflower seeds, and walnuts
Iron	Red meats, chicken and turkey, liver, green vegetables, and dried fruits
Vitamin C	Tomatoes, berries, citrus fruits, and green vegetables
Zinc	Red meat, oysters, nuts, seeds, and whole grains

Several natural or herbal therapies have been used to reduce hair loss and thinning, and promote healthy hair growth. However, most of these have not been assessed by proper scientific studies so their efficacy is really unknown. They are all thought to work by reducing the conversion of testosterone to DHT.

Examples of these are:

- Green tea
- Saw palmetto
- Stinging nettle.

However, even though these products are considered 'natural', if they are potent enough to cause a hormonal change in the body then they are potent enough to cause side effects in some women. You really should see a reputable herbalist or clinical nutritionist who can assess you, discuss the most suitable treatments for you, prescribe the appropriate doses, and monitor you. He/she can also advise you where to buy the supplements as unfortunately there is wide variation in the quality of over-the-counter nutritional and herbal supplements.

What your doctor can do

You may be devastated by your hair loss. You may feel unfeminine and unattractive. Do go and see your doctor who will be able to rule out other common causes for your hair loss such as thyroid disease or iron deficiency. Your doctor can then refer you to a skin specialist, or dermatologist, who can assess you, confirm that it is androgenic alopecia, or male-pattern hair thinning related to PCOS, and discuss the treatment options with you (Table 11.3). The earlier you start treatment, the more effective the treatment is likely to be. However, remember there is no cure for hair loss. Treatments may improve hair thinning, but hair loss usually recurs when medication is stopped.

Summary

Hair thinning is an uncommon but distressing symptom of PCOS caused by an increased sensitivity of the hair follicles on the scalp to androgens. The good news is that it rarely progresses to baldness. A well-balanced nutritious diet is important for healthy hair. There are treatments available which do reduce hair loss and encourage hair regrowth, although they are not suitable for, or effective in, everyone. Treatment is most effective the earlier it is started, so if you are concerned about hair thinning then do see your doctor. A combination of topical minoxidil and an anti-androgen may produce the best results. Hair thinning does recur if treatment is stopped.

Table 11.3 Medical treatments for hair loss in PCOS

	Side effects	Notes
Minoxidil 2% solution Minoxidil (Regaine) applied directly to the scalp twice a day stimulates hair growth. No one knows exactly how minoxidil stimulates hair growth	◆ May result in increased facial hair growth at the higher dose ◆ The amount of minoxidil absorbed through the skin into the bloodstream is usually too small to cause other significant side effects	◆ Causes mild to moderate hair regrowth in about 50% of women and slows down hair loss in up to 90% of users. It is most effective if started early. It takes at least 3–6 months to see any benefit but if there has been no change by 6 months then it is unlikely to work ◆ Clinical trials have shown that 5% (extra strength) minoxidil is significantly more effective in both retaining and regrowing hair in women than the 2% solution. However, in the UK the 5% solution is only available for men ◆ Minoxidil is unavailable on an NHS prescription. It is expensive, costing about £25 a month, and if you stop using it unfortunately the hair loss tends to recur
Anti-androgens e.g. spironolactone, cyproterone acetate, and flutamide Reduce the production of androgens by the ovaries and block the action of androgens on the skin	◆ All anti-androgens must be taken with contraception as they can be harmful to the unborn fetus ◆ See Table 10.2 for full list of side effects and precautions	◆ Spironolactone and cyproterone acetate have been used to treat male-pattern hair thinning in women with PCOS with varying degrees of success, and are best used to minimize further hair loss. However, they are not licensed to be used to treat hair loss ◆ Flutamide has been shown to result in modest hair regrowth in women. However, it is rarely used in the UK as it has been associated with fatal liver disease

(continued)

Table 11.3 Medical treatments for hair loss in PCOS *(continued)*

	Side effects	Notes
Combined oral contraceptive pill Dianette contains a small dose of cyproterone acetate while Yasmin contains a substance similar to spironolactone	◆ Nausea, breast tenderness, mood disturbances, weight gain, reduced libido, and an increased risk of blood clots ◆ Do not use if: • you have previously had a blood clot • you are over the age of 35 years and are a smoker or are overweight • you have high blood pressure or migraines	◆ Dianette has been used to treat androgenic alopecia with some effect. The efficacy of Yasmin on hair thinning is still unknown as it is a relatively new drug
Finasteride Prevents testosterone from being converted into the more active androgen DHT	◆ It can interfere with development of the baby's genitals if the baby in the womb is male. In fact, if you are pregnant or are thinking of becoming pregnant, it is advised that you should not even touch a finasteride tablet	◆ It is taken as a once-daily tablet ◆ Appears to be at least as effective as Regaine in men. There has only been one small study in women, with encouraging results. Not licensed in women but your dermatologist or endocrinologist may prescribe it as long as you take reliable contraception and you are monitored regularly. It takes about 3–6 months to see an effect and has to be taken indefinitely if hair growth is to continue. Studies suggest that the longer it is taken, the thicker and longer the hairs become. Men have continued to take it for 5 years with good results. However, as with all treatments listed above, as soon as medication is stopped hair loss recurs

12

The treatment of acne

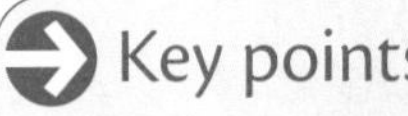

- About 25% of women with PCOS develop acne.
- Acne is a very treatable condition and many women will see some improvement using over-the-counter medicated cleansers.
- If your skin is still very inflamed then your doctor may prescribe stronger topical treatments and/ or antibiotics. A minority of women will not respond and will need to be referred to a skin specialist for further treatment.

About 1 in 4 women with PCOS are troubled with greasy skin, spots, and acne well after their teenage years. The good news is that acne is usually treatable, although you may need treatment for several years to keep the spots at bay.

I had never suffered from spots as a teenager, but in my late twenties I started to get spots that were very red and painful on my face, shoulders and back.

What causes acne?

Acne is inflammation of the oil glands of the skin on the face, back, and chest. Remember that each hair follicle has an oil gland known as the sebaceous gland connected to it (Fig. 12.1). Oil, or sebum, is normally secreted through the pore of the hair follicle to keep skin and hair in good condition. In general, the more sebum you produce, the greasier your skin and the more likely you are to develop spots or acne. Sebum production is under the influence

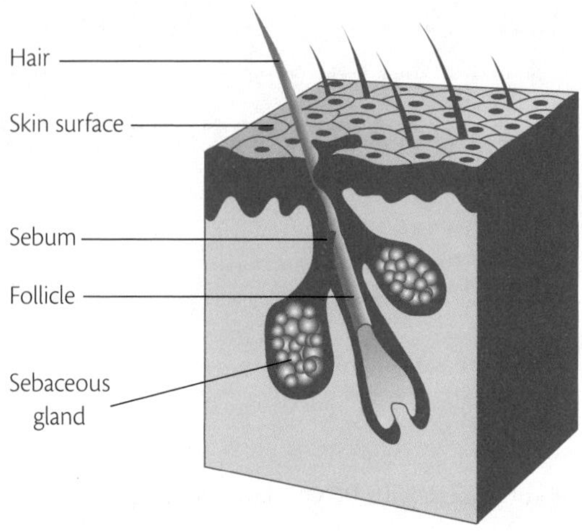

Figure 12.1 The hair follicle and sebaceous glands.

of androgens, particularly testosterone. People who suffer from acne tend to have sebaceous glands which are more sensitive to testosterone and secrete more sebum than they should. Women with PCOS also often have higher levels of free testosterone than usual, compounding the problem. Spots then develop if the pores through which the hairs emerge become partially blocked by dead skin cells shed into the pore. This results in tiny spots (comedones), known as whiteheads or blackheads, and is considered mild acne. The black of the blackheads is skin pigment and not dirt. If the pore becomes completely blocked, the oil builds up around the hair root and becomes infected with bacteria normally present on the skin. This causes inflammation, resulting in redness, pus formation, and pain—the spot or pimple. In many cases there is no further progression beyond mild to moderate acne.

In more severe cases the pus caused by the bacterial infection bursts deep into the skin rather than onto the surface. This results in pustules and even cyst formation. When pustules and cysts eventually heal, scarring may occur. Scars are usually permanent, and so it is important to treat acne early not only to minimize the psychological distress often associated with symptoms that effect your appearance but also to prevent scarring.

Myths about acne

Myth: Acne is caused by dirt or poor cleanliness

Fact: Acne is caused by excess sebum production and blockage of the skin pores, usually in response to sensitivity to testosterone. Wash your face using mild soap and water about twice a day. Washing it excessively will dry the skin up and have little effect on the spots. Do not scrub your skin as this may cause more inflammation and make the acne worse.

Myth: Acne is due to eating too much sugar or fried food

Fact: Although you should have a healthy diet, fatty or sugary foods do not cause acne.

Myth: Acne is contagious

Fact: Although there is a build-up of bacteria in the sebum of blocked pores causing the inflammation, the bacteria are found normally on the skin.

Myth: Squeezing the spots can help clear up acne

Fact: Squeezing spots can actually help spread the infection and can cause inflammation and a tendency to scarring.

What can make acne worse?

- Excessive sweating. For example, humid climates or working in very hot environments can cause acne to flare up. The excessive sweating may block the pores.
- Some medication. Steroids, some anti-epilepsy drugs, and progesterone-only contraceptives (minipill) can make acne worse. If you think that medicines you are taking have made your acne worse, you should speak to your doctor, but never stop medication without medical advice.
- Premenstrually. Many women notice that their acne gets worse about a week before their period starts. This is due to monthly changes in hormone levels.

- Certain beauty products. Greasy or thick foundation may exacerbate acne by blocking pores. However, most make-up should not affect acne. Try using oil-free moisturizers if possible. Also, some hair oils, wax, or serum used to prevent frizzy hair may induce spots along the hair margin.
- Stress may cause an exacerbation of acne in some people.

When should I see my doctor?

Do not be embarrassed about seeing your doctor about your acne. Acne can be emotionally distressing as it affects your appearance. However, acne is a very treatable condition. We would suggest that you try over-the-counter medicated cleansers such as Clearasil, Clean and Clear Cleansing Lotion, or Neutrogena Clear Pore Lotion. If these do not work, then you could try benzoyl peroxide cream or gel (Table 12.1), but if you have not seen a difference in your skin within 8 weeks you should see your GP who can prescribe other treatments. If you have large tender pimples or pustules then you should consider seeing your doctor sooner as more aggressive treatment may need to be started early to prevent scarring. If you are dark skinned and develop dark patches where the spots used to be you should also seek medical advice. If you have severe acne your doctor may even refer you to a dermatologist (skin specialist).

How long will I need treatment for acne?

Treatment takes at least 8–12 weeks before significant improvement is seen, and you may need treatment for at least 6 months, and often several years, to prevent acne from recurring. When you stop treatment you may have a flare-up of acne so you may need topical treatments for several years to keep the acne under control.

Natural treatments for acne

There is some anecdotal evidence that some herbs and nutrients may help improve acne, but there is no widespread clinical evidence that they will definitely help.

- Aloe vera gel and tea tree oil are good treatments for acne as they have antibacterial properties. Just dab a little on the spots.
- Vitamin B_6 can help to regulate male and female hormones levels, which may improve acne.
- Zinc may reduce inflammation and may help balance hormone levels, thereby reducing sebum production.

Table 12.1 Treatment options for acne

	Mechanism of action	**Side effects**	**Notes**
Topical (applied directly to the skin)			
Benzoyl peroxide	Kills bacteria and unblocks the pores, allowing the sebum to drain.	◆ Skin irritation and dryness. Use the lowest strength first to minimize skin irritation and wash off after a few hours. Gradually increase the amount of time you keep the solution on your skin, aiming to apply it twice a day. Creams are less drying than gels but you should use a good oil-free moisturiser ◆ Can bleach hair, clothes, and other fabrics, so wash off immediately if fabrics or your hair come into contact with it.	◆ Can be bought without a prescription ◆ Available as a gel, cream, and face wash in different strengths. Ask your pharmacist for advice on products ◆ Mild acne (a few whiteheads and blackheads) can be treated with benzoyl peroxide alone. If after 8 weeks there has been little improvement then you should see your doctor and consider additional treatments ◆ Benzoyl peroxide may be used in moderate or severe acne in combination with other treatments.
Azelaic acid	Kills bacteria and unblocks pores	◆ Less likely to irritate the skin ◆ Azelaic acid may harm the fetus, so you must not use during pregnancy or if you are considering becoming pregnant	◆ Requires a prescription ◆ It is useful for treating mild acne but should not be used for more than 6 months

(continued)

Table 12.1 Treatment options for acne *(continued)*

	Mechanism of action	Side effects	Notes
Retinoids	These are vitamin A derivatives which act by helping unblock pores	◆ Often cause skin dryness and an increased tendency to sunburn, so you must use a good sunblock and a good moisturizer ◆ Your skin may go red and start peeling when you first start using a retinoid, but this usually settles with time ◆ Retinoids may harm the fetus so you must not use during pregnancy or if you are considering becoming pregnant	◆ There are several brands available, in cream or gel form, but only by a doctor's prescription ◆ They can be very useful in the treatment of blackheads and whiteheads
Antibiotics e.g. clindamycin, erythromycin	Kill bacteria and are particularly useful if there is inflammation	◆ Do not cause as much irritation as the other solutions.	◆ Antibiotics in gel, lotion, or solution form are available on prescription. Should be used for at least 6 months for maximum benefit. Often as effective as taking antibiotics by mouth ◆ They do not unblock pores, so unless they are combined with benzoyl peroxide, blackheads and whiteheads may remain

Tablets			
Antibiotics e.g. tetracycline, doxycycline, eryrthromycin	Kill the bacteria and reduce inflammation	◆ You must let your doctor know if you are pregnant or are considering pregnancy as some antibiotics should not be taken during pregnancy	◆ Can be prescribed for moderate to severe acne, often in combination with a topical solution such as benzoyl peroxide ◆ It takes about 6 weeks for antibiotics to work so do not give up after a week or two. If there has been little improvement after 3 months then see your doctor who may prescribe a different antibiotic. Maximum improvement takes up to 6 months but many women may need 1–2 years of treatment
Combined oral contraceptive pill	Reduces the effect of testosterone on sebum production	◆ Nausea, breast tenderness, mood disturbances, weight gain, reduced libido, and an increased risk of blood clots ◆ Do not use if: • you have previously had a blood clot • you are over the age of 35 years and are a smoker or are overweight • you have high blood pressure or migraines	◆ Dianette is a contraceptive pill which contains a male hormone blocker, cyproterone acetate. It is as effective as antibiotics but you may need topical treatments as well ◆ Yasmin is another contraceptive pill which contains drospirenone and causes less weight gain than Dianette ◆ Yasmin is a relatively new drug so we do not know whether it is as effective as Dianette in treating acne ◆ Other male hormone blockers such as spironolactone may also help acne

(continued)

Table 12.1 Treatment options for acne *(continued)*

	Mechanism of action	Side effects	Notes
Isotretinoin (Roaccutane)	Reduces sebum production Very effective and often a permanent cure for acne	◆ The most common side effect is dryness of the skin ◆ Can cause serious side effects such as liver damage, visual problems, depression, mood disturbances, and high blood fat levels ◆ A pregnancy test has to be done before starting treatment and you must be on contraception as it is very toxic to the fetus. You will need regular blood tests to monitor your liver function and blood fats while on isoretinoin	◆ Can only be used to treat severe acne if other treatments have not worked and can only be prescribed by a dermatologist (skin specialist). This is because it is very toxic

- Essential fatty acids, or omega-3 and omega-6, may reduce inflammation, and the risk of pores becoming clogged and spots developing.
- The herbs chasteberry (also known as *Vitex agnus-castus*) and dong quai may also balance your hormone levels, improving the appearance of acne.

Even though these products are considered 'natural', if they are potent enough to cause a hormonal change in the body then they are potent enough to cause side effects in some women. You should really see a medical nutritionist or herbalist who can advise you on the best preparations for you. It is important that you see a reputable nutritionist, someone who is recommended by a friend, or someone who is registered with a professional body. He/she can assess you, prescribe the appropriate doses, and monitor you. Your nutritionist or herbalist can also advise you where to buy the supplements as unfortunately there is wide variation in the quality of over-the-counter nutritional and herbal supplements.

Treatment of scarring

Acne can result in permanent scarring if it is severe and left untreated. The scars can initially be red or purple in colour but the colour disappears over 1–2 years. However, you may be left with deep pock marks. Laser treatment, abrasion, and chemical peels can help, but the skin rarely returns completely to normal. These techniques remove the top layers of skin, resulting in a smoother appearance. It is best to discuss the treatments and success rates with your skin specialist (dermatologist). They are not without their side effects or risks. The treated area of skin may remain pink, sensitive, and swollen for several weeks after treatment, and in some cases the technique itself can cause scarring, particularly if you have dark skin. It may take up to a year to see the full results of treatment.

Patient's perspective

Nicola, aged 27 years, had had bad acne on her back and face since she was 17 years old. She had tried various course of antibiotics but the spots came back a few months after stopping the treatment. She then went onto Dianette and after a few months of being on it, she had really clear skin. She stopped the Dianette following 5 years of treatment and her skin remains clear.

Part 3

Weight management in polycystic ovary syndrome

Introduction

By the time the majority of women with PCOS get round to attending a specialist clinic, they have usually tried every single 'diet' there is. These women will report either that the diet 'didn't work' or that they lost a couple of stone before putting that couple of stone back on along with a little bit more. The following chapters aim to remove the myths about losing weight and give you the information you need to lose weight and, most importantly, to keep it off.

13

Before you begin to try to lose weight

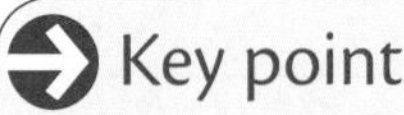

- In order to lose weight you must be motivated to do so. Your level of motivation may be constantly changing.
- It is important to attempt to lose weight only when you are ready to commit to making changes to your eating and activity behaviour.
- The symptoms of PCOS may be significantly improved by losing just 5% of your body weight.

People who try half-heartedly to lose weight are unlikely to succeed. In fact, a half-hearted attempt at losing weight might even to do more harm than good. Success breeds success, and vice versa, and trying to lose weight without succeeding may reduce the amount of confidence you have that you can lose weight in the future.

In order to be successful at losing weight, you must be able to put time and effort into changing your behaviour—no one else can do it for you. If you are in the middle of a crisis at home or at work, it is unlikely that you will be able to focus on making these changes. It is therefore much more sensible to put it off until you are ready to give it your full attention.

Why don't diets work?

When the word 'diet' is entered as a keyword in the search bar on Amazon.com, we are presented with around 190 000 book titles, all of which aim to help improve our current diets and the majority of which are designed to help us lose weight. With so many supposedly effective methods available to lose weight, we should be surprised that the UK population continues to become heavier and heavier. It has been estimated that, out of 100 people who are trying to lose weight, only between one and five will manage to lose 5 per cent or more of their starting body weight and keep it off for a year. A much greater percentage will manage to lose the weight; the main problem appears to be keeping it off. So why is it that diets don't work? When we put this question to the women attending our PCOS clinic, these are some of the most common answers.

Because there is too much temptation everywhere from tasty high-calorie foods.

Because diets make me feel deprived so I think about [naughty] foods all the time.

Because I go out a lot and the rules of the diets don't fit in with that.

I always start off well but I run out of willpower.

Certainly nearly all popular diets provide the reader with a novel set of rules to follow in order to lose weight. They separate foods into two groups—'good' and 'bad'—with some even referring to higher-calorie foods as 'sins'. This simply serves to increase our guilt after eating one of these forbidden foods. This guilt then inevitably results in us eating even more of the offending food, in an effort to get the craving out of our system so that we can 'start again tomorrow' with none of that 'bad' food.

What diets don't take account of is the emotional side of eating. We don't merely eat when we are hungry; we eat when we are stressed, bored, or simply because others are eating so we like to be sociable and join in.

Women are often given unrealistic expectations by magazine articles and advertisements, which bombard us with headlines about 'losing 10 pounds in a week' or dropping four clothes sizes in a matter of months. We put a huge amount of effort into trying to lose weight, and we become very despondent when we lose weight at a slower rate than these articles suggest we should. The point at which the dieter becomes disappointed with their weight loss is usually the point at which all willpower vanishes.

The more experienced dieters will have no doubt already come to the conclusion that any weight loss is good and that this time they really need to modify their lifestyle for the long term rather than go on yet another 'diet'. However, to most people, this can sound like an even more daunting prospect. By telling ourselves that we are going to change to 'healthy eating' or 'a healthier lifestyle', what we are really thinking is 'this means I have to eat less chocolate and crisps for ever'. This can lead to even greater feelings of deprivation than a quick-fix 'diet' would have produced.

It is important to bear in mind that diets only teach people how to lose weight. They do not teach people the incredibly important new skills that are needed to keep weight the same once weight loss has been achieved. The aim of this book is not to help you lose the largest amount of weight in the shortest possible time. Its aim is to remove the mystery surrounding weight management and to provide you with the information and skills you may need in the longer term, so that you no longer need to battle with your weight.

Are you motivated enough?

You must be motivated in order to succeed at losing weight. You will probably think of this motivation as simply the desire to be slimmer, i.e. how **important** losing weight is to you. However, the other, equally important, aspect of motivation is the amount of **confidence** you have that there is something you can do to change the way you are (see Figure 13.1). Even if you really do want to lose weight, it will be difficult for you to do so if you don't believe that you can.

How **important** weight loss is to you depends on two things.

- Your knowledge

  For example:

  - Your own knowledge that losing weight will improve your symptoms
  - Your own knowledge of the risk to your health of being overweight
  - Your own knowledge about the shape and size you would like to be

- Your concern

  For example:

  - To what extent your own symptoms of PCOS bother you
  - To what extent it worries you that your health is at risk because you are overweight
  - To what extent it concerns you that you are not the shape or size you would like to be.

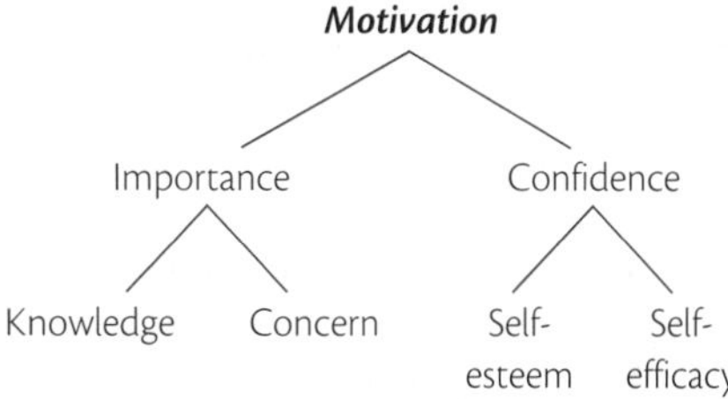

Figure 13.1 The components of motivation.

How **confident** you are that you can lose weight also depends on two things.

- Your self-esteem
  - How much value you place on yourself—your self-worth
  - How much you believe that you deserve to be happy
- Your self-efficacy
  - The extent to which you believe that there is something you can do which will help you achieve your goals
  - The extent to which you believe that if you try you will succeed

It is important to remember that none of these factors stay the same. The amount of knowledge you have about weight and losing weight will increase as you find out more about it. How concerned you are about your weight will change according to the severity of your symptoms and other weight-related health problems. Your level of concern might also change according to changes in the behaviour of people around you. I know several women whose most successful attempts at weight loss were triggered when a stranger gave up their seat on the train in the mistaken belief that they were pregnant. Your self-esteem and self-efficacy may vary immensely according to other aspects of your life, such as personal relationships or successes at work. It is not uncommon for women with PCOS to have very low self-esteem. This is no surprise, as all the symptoms of PCOS can make women feel less attractive and less feminine than women without PCOS. It is therefore possible that, by treating a symptom such as unwanted hair, you may improve your self-esteem and, in turn, your motivation to lose weight.

> To my horror, she looked at me and said 'How fantastic—you're pregnant!'
>
> 'No, I'm just fat', I calmly replied.

So, even if you do not have the motivation to lose weight right now, it does not mean that you will never have that motivation. This is important to bear in mind, especially if you are someone who says:

I can't lose weight, I just don't have the willpower.

The cycle of change

There are several stages in the cycle of change (Prochaska and Di Clemente[1] 1986) as shown in Fig. 13.2.

[1] Prochaska, J.O., DiClemente, C.C., *et al.*: Self-change of psychological distress: laypersons' vs. psychologists' coping strategies. *Journal of Clinical Psychology* (1986) Sep; **42**(5): 834–40.

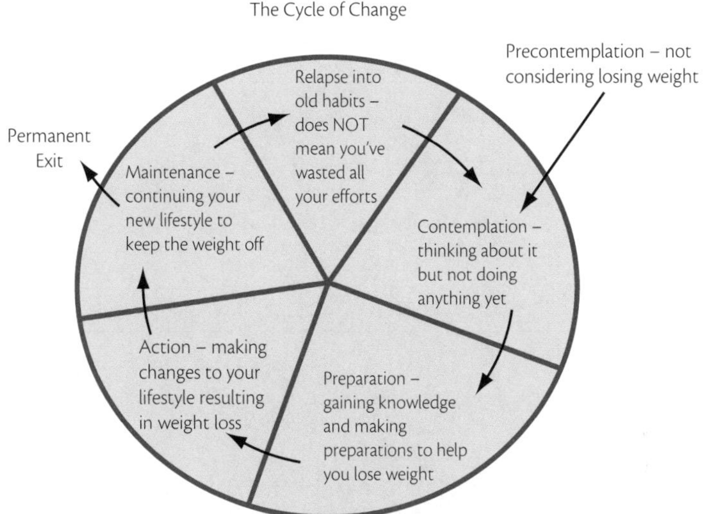

Figure 13.2 The cycle of change (based on the model by Prochaska and Di Clemente, 1986). Reproduced with kind permission of Professor Prochaska.

As you are reading this book, it is likely that you are already at the preparation stage. You might, however, be reading it because you've just been told you have PCOS and are only just discovering that your weight has a major impact on this condition. For the majority of readers, you will have been battling with your weight for as long as you can remember, so you are already at the action stage, but find it difficult to remain motivated and so end up relapsing too often, resulting in no weight loss or even weight gain.

Ambivalence

It is very common for women attending the PCOS clinic to say things like this.

- I know I should try to eat breakfast everyday, but I just don't have time in the mornings.
- I know I shouldn't buy so many biscuits and crisps, but I've got to because my husband and children need them.
- I know I shouldn't eat take-aways so often, but I'm just so hungry when I get back from work and I haven't got time to cook.

Table 13.1 The pros and cons of changing

	Pros	Cons
Making changes to your lifestyle to enable you to lose weight		
Not making any changes to your lifestyle and continuing as you are (think about how you will feel in 6 months time)		

Saying 'Yes, but ...' about making a change to your behaviour implies that you are in two minds about making that change. Filling in Table 13.1 might help you decide what you really want. Fill it in for yourself, including as many points in each box as you feel apply to you. When you have filled in the table as completely as possible, read the whole thing back to yourself.

If the benefits of making changes to your lifestyle do not outweigh the effort required to do so, it is perhaps not the right time for you to be trying to lose weight. You should therefore wait until you are able to make the changes required. If you do have the desire to lose weight (the benefits of losing weight outweigh the effort required to do so), the following chapters will give you the confidence that indeed you **can** lose weight.

Expectations of weight loss

In order that you succeed in achieving your weight loss goals, it is extremely important that these goals are realistic and attainable. Success breeds success, so you are likely to go on succeeding at losing weight if you set yourself manageable targets. See the two case studies below to see why realistic targets are so important.

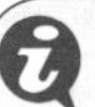

Patients' perspectives

Maria was 15 stone on New Year's Day and wanted to be 10 stone by her sister's wedding in March. She went on a strict diet, and completely cut out all the biscuits and cakes she used to eat between meals. She also walked for 30 minutes each day. She started to lose weight at an average rate of 1 lb per week. By March, having been on her diet for 14 weeks, she had lost a stone. She realized then that it was very unlikely that she would lose another 4 stone by the wedding day, so she gave up completely and went back to her old habits. By May she had regained the stone she had lost.

Kristina was 15 stone on New Year's Day and wanted to lose weight for her sister's wedding in March. She understood that, if she reduced her calorie intake by eating fewer biscuits between meals and reducing the fat content of her meals, she might be able to lose about 1 lb per week. She acknowledged that it was her birthday in February so she might not have been able to lose weight around that time. She decided she would aim to be 10 lb lighter by her sister's wedding. On the morning of the wedding, Kristina stepped onto the scales and was delighted to see that she was 14 stone 2 lb—a loss of 12 lb. After the wedding, she continued with her lower-calorie diet, and by June she had lost 2 stone.

As you can see from these stories, setting yourself a small target that you know you can achieve is likely to help you to lose more weight in the long term. Setting yourself an unrealistic, unachievable target may cause your weight to yo-yo and is likely to result in weight gain over the longer term.

How much weight should you expect to lose?

Experts in weight management regard 'success' as managing to lose 5 per cent of your starting body weight and keeping it off. Furthermore, several studies have reported that a loss of 5 per cent of starting body weight can significantly improve the symptoms of PCOS. However, studies have shown that only between 1 and 5 per cent of people who are trying to lose weight manage to maintain weight loss of 5 per cent, or, to put it another way, 95–99 per cent fail to lose this 5 per cent and keep it off. If you have ever lost weight and then regained it, one of the reasons for this may have been that you wanted to lose more than 5 per cent of your body weight. You would then have been disappointed when you had 'only' lost 5 per cent. You might have thought 'What's the point in carrying on?' and gone back to your old habits, regaining all the weight you had lost. It is not just the people who are trying to lose weight who have unrealistic expectations—your doctor may have told you that 'you need to lose four stone to get down to your ideal weight'. This will only result in your being disappointed and frustrated when you fail to lose this unachievable amount of weight.

So you're telling me that I'm only likely to lose a stone or so, but I need to lose at least four!

For someone who is 15 stone 12 lb, losing 5 per cent of their body weight means losing 11 lb. However, most people who are 15 stone 12 lb find it difficult to accept that they have been successful when they get down to 15 stone 1 lb.

Another reason why people tend to give up and revert back to their old habits is that they expect weight to come off steadily. It is perfectly normal to lose, for example, 2 lb in the first week, nothing the second week, and 1 lb the next week. This indicates that you are losing 1 lb of fat per week with normal fluctuations in fluid weight. Unfortunately, many people would have given up completely after week 2 when the scales showed no weight loss in return for their efforts.

How long should you expect to lose weight for?

Studies have shown that most people will only be able to lose weight for 12–15 weeks before they reach a plateau. Many people believe that this is because their metabolic rate decreases when they lose weight. However, this reduction in metabolic rate is small. The main reason for the plateau is that people's motivation and enthusiasm for losing weight begin to lag, so they begin to consume more calories and expend fewer calories through exercise than they were when they were losing weight more rapidly.

Therefore, to keep your goals realistic, you should be aiming to lose 5 per cent of your body weight in 12–15 weeks; then you should aim to keep your weight the same (i.e. not gaining weight but not actively trying to lose it) for at least a month. After maintaining your new lower weight for a while, you may then find that you're ready to try to lose another 5 per cent. This way you are likely to lose more over the longer term.

What else can you expect from weight loss?

It is common for people to expect other aspects of their lives to change as a result of losing weight.

It may be that someone wants to lose weight:

(1) to reduce their unwanted hair growth and improve their fertility

(2) so that they feel more attractive

(3) so that they can land their dream job.

These are their **primary goals** and losing weight is, in their eyes, the stepping stone to achieving them. Is it very important that your primary goals are realistic in the same way that your weight loss goals must be realistic. We know that losing 5 per cent of your body weight is likely to reduce your insulin and testosterone levels and therefore reduce the symptoms of PCOS. Therefore it is possible to achieve the first goal through weight loss, though other factors should be considered at the same time, such as medications and cosmetic treatments. The second and third goals, however, involve many other factors as well as weight, so they may not be achieved simply through losing a realistic 5 per cent of your body weight. It is always worth pursuing these primary goals at the same time as trying to lose weight; for example, having a haircut, trying out new clothes styles and make-up, and being more active can help you feel more attractive even before you have reached your target weight. Too often we put off doing important things until we have lost weight, and this can further reduce our self-esteem and self-efficacy, which in turn actually hinders our ability to lose the weight.

14

What should you be eating?

Key points

- A healthy balanced diet is one which provides all the nutrients required for good health in the appropriate amounts for each individual.
- Sitting down to three tasty, balanced meals per day helps you to eat a balanced diet and reduces the likelihood of grazing on less nutritious, high-calorie snacks.
- Alcohol intake should not exceed 2–3 units per day, as higher intakes are damaging to health and may result in a higher calorie intake.

A balanced diet

With so many books and articles about 'healthy eating' and 'dieting', and with many of these articles being based on the latest celebrity food fads, it can be difficult to know which of the conflicting pieces of advice to believe. A healthy balanced diet should follow the recommendations made by the Department of Health as set out in advice from the Food Standards Agency and large professional organizations such as the British Dietetic Association. Figure 14.1 depicts the gold standard for a healthy diet in terms of the proportions that the different food groups should make up. There are no 'good' and 'bad' foods and you are encouraged to eat every type of food that you like. It is the proportions of the various foods that are important.

However much an individual needs to eat to keep in good health, the proportions that the various food groups make up in the diet should remain the same. So, for example, a 60 kg woman who is a competitive triathlete will require proportionately larger quantities of **all** the food groups than a 60 kg woman of the same age who has a sedentary lifestyle. Even though the triathlete's calorie

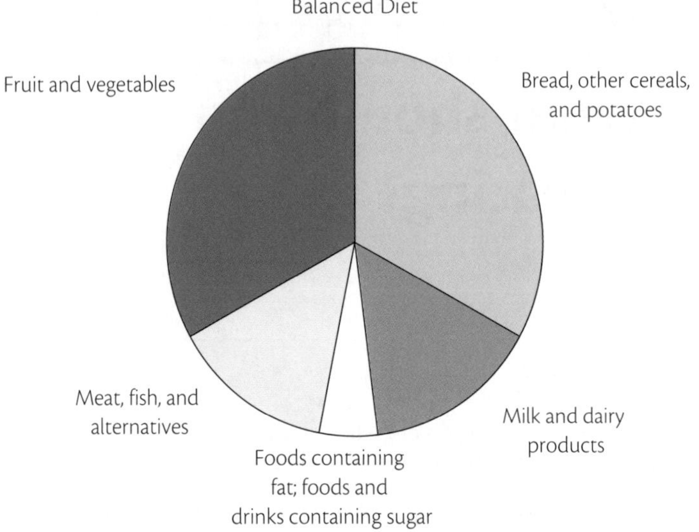

Figure 14.1 A balanced diet.

intake would be much greater to meet her increased requirements, the overall balance of her diet should be just the same.

The four main food groups are:

- Bread, other cereals and potatoes
- Fruit and vegetables
- Meat, fish and alternatives
- Milk and dairy products

The fifth food group is 'Foods containing fat; foods and drinks containing sugar'. These are included in a healthy balanced diet, as they are tasty, but, as they are high in calories and have little value nutritionally, they should be eaten sparingly.

Bread, other cereals and potatoes

This group includes all bread, chapattis, cereals, oats, pasta, rice, noodles, potatoes, and sweet potatoes, and dishes made from yam, plantain, bulgar wheat, maize, and cornmeal.

These foods should form a major part of each meal, as they are nutritious and filling, and high-fibre varieties can help maintain a healthy digestive system. Remember that these are the nutritional guidelines for the population as a whole and that, by manipulating their carbohydrate intake, women with PCOS may find it easier to lose weight. This is not because these starchy foods are 'fattening' but because many women with PCOS tend to overeat these foods, for example eating excessive amounts of bread as between-meal snacks. We also often add a high-fat accompaniment to the foods in this group—for example eating butter or margarine with bread and potatoes, or olive oil on pasta.

Fruits and vegetables

This group includes all fresh, frozen, dried, and tinned fruit and vegetables. Beans, pulses, and fruit juice may also account for up to one portion per day.

We should all be eating at least five portions of foods from this group per day, with one portion being roughly equivalent to one large handful (about 80 g). The reason for this is that people who eat more fruit and vegetables are much less likely to suffer from heart disease, stroke, or cancer. Given that women with PCOS are at much higher risk of cardiovascular disease than women without PCOS, it is even more important that you eat your five-a-day. The protective health effects of fruit and vegetables are not simply down to the antioxidant vitamins they contain, so the same protection cannot be obtained by taking a multivitamin supplement. Fruits and vegetables are usually low in calories and so are a good way to fill yourself up if you are trying to lose weight—an average apple contains about 60 calories while an average biscuit contains about 80 calories (and who eats just one biscuit?!?). When serving your main meal of the day, aim to fill half your plate with vegetables. Try making soups, casseroles, and stir-fries as a good way to include a larger variety of interesting and tasty vegetables.

Milk and dairy foods

This group includes milk, cheeses, yoghurts, and fromage frais. We need these foods because they are the best source of calcium in the diet, which is essential for strong bones and to prevent osteoporosis (brittle bones) in later life. However, many people who are trying to lose weight appear virtually to cut out dairy products, perceiving them to be 'fattening'. It is important to remember that skimmed and semi-skimmed milks contain just as much calcium as whole milk, so by choosing low-fat dairy products you will be getting enough calcium without taking in a large number of calories.

Cooked dishes made from lower-fat milk, such as sauces, custards, and milky puddings, also provide calcium.

Meat, fish, and alternatives

This group includes all types of meat and fish as well as eggs, beans, pulses, nuts, and meat substitutes such as soya protein products and Quorn.

They are the main source of protein in the diet and are a good source of iron. Most people eat more protein than they really need and many protein foods are high in fat as well as protein, so it is worth keeping portion sizes small and choosing lower-fat types. Lower-fat types include lean cuts of meat with visible fat removed, fish, eggs, beans, pulses, and meat substitutes. Some manufactured products may have a lot of added fat, so watch out for this in sausages, pies, burgers, and pâtés.

The Department of Health recommends that we include fish in the diet, particularly oily fish, which has been shown to be protective against heart disease. The number of servings recommended for protection against heart disease is 2–3 per week. If you are not planning on having any children, then you may eat up to four portions of oily fish per week; however, due to concerns over toxins which accumulate in fish, women of childbearing age should not eat more than two portions of oily fish per week.

Foods containing fat; foods and drinks containing sugar

A balanced diet also consists of a fifth group which includes:

- All fats and oils (including low-fat spreads and oils perceived to be 'healthy')
- Mayonnaise, cream, and other high-fat dressings and dips
- Pastries, pies, pasties
- Crisps and other deep-fried snacks such as mini spring rolls, samosas, etc.
- Sweets, chocolate, cakes, biscuits, and sweet desserts
- Sugar and sugary drinks (squashes and fizzy drinks containing sugar).

Everyone eats indulgence foods such as chocolate, biscuits, crisps, sweets, and cakes, but these foods are not particularly nutritious and they are a very dense source of calories. They are usually eaten for pleasure, not for their nutritional contribution to the diet. Although it is true that we do need some fat in our diet to prevent deficiency and to make our food palatable, the amount required is so small that it is not necessary for us to eat high-fat foods to meet our bodies' requirement. Sugar serves no useful nutritional purpose; it simply provides calories and sweetness, nothing else. Therefore, we can consider sugar to provide 'empty calories'. It is recommended that we eat foods containing fat, and foods and drinks containing sugar, sparingly, so these foods should be kept as occasional treats. If you think you are eating too many foods from this group, you can try to reduce this amount by looking at how you are eating them.

- Frequency—could you have chocolate twice a week instead of four times a week?
- Amount—could you serve yourself two biscuits on a plate instead of munching them freely with the packet by your side?
- Type—could you choose reduced-fat mayonnaise instead of ordinary mayonnaise?

As a very general guide, Table 14.1 may help you work out whether the amount of fat, sugar, and saturated fat listed on food labels is a little or a lot.

Table 14.1 A little and a lot—per 100 g of a food

A LITTLE means:	2 g sugars 3 g fat 1 g saturated fat	or LESS
A LOT means:	10 g sugars 20 g fat 5 g saturated fat	or MORE

For more information on labelling, see www.eatwell.gov.uk

Many of the foods in this group are indulgence foods, and people often use these as a treat or reward or as a comfort. In addition, women with PCOS are more likely to experience strong cravings for sugary foods as a result of their high insulin levels. See Chapter 18 for more information about PCOS, carbohydrates, and insulin, and to find out how to choose sensible carbohydrates at mealtimes to help reduce your carbohydrate cravings.

It is very difficult to eat less of these high-sugar high-fat foods if you are eating them for emotional reasons, especially if eating them then makes you feel guilty. Try some of the techniques in Chapter 20 to help you gain control over your consumption of these foods.

Meal pattern

As well as placing emphasis on the types of foods we should eat, it is important to remember that, in order for someone to eat a healthy diet and to lose weight, they must establish a regular eating pattern. Studies have consistently shown that people who skip meals find it harder to control their weight than people who eat at regular intervals. Someone who has a regular meal pattern usually eats what they consider to be 'proper meals', which provide them with the nutrients their body needs, rather than continuously grazing on foods with little nutritional value. Furthermore, people who take the time to sit down to proper meals find their food more satisfying than people who graze throughout the day. If you skip meals, you will inevitably end up snacking on more high-fat high-sugar foods. This may be for a number of reasons, which are explained in Chapters 20 and 23. Certainly it may be easier to adhere to healthy eating recommendations if you eat regular meals including breakfast.

Salt

Salt is the common name for sodium chloride. We all need some sodium in our diet, but most of us have consumed the whole of our daily requirement by the time we have finished our breakfast. About 75 per cent of the salt in our diets comes from processed foods, so we may well be eating too much even if we do not add any at the table or in cooking. Eating too much sodium can lead to high blood pressure, which is a risk factor for stroke and heart disease. The government's recommendations are that adults should have no more than 6 g of salt per day (equivalent to 2.5 g of sodium). However, it is important to bear in mind that, if you are overweight and have high blood pressure, losing weight is by far the best way to reduce your blood pressure. Therefore, even if a food is low in salt, it does not mean that it is necessarily a healthy option for you.

For example, if you had high blood pressure and were overweight, which would you choose out of the following two spreads:

- unsalted butter
- ordinary reduced-fat margarine.

Well, the butter, despite being lower in salt, is still extremely high in fat and calories, whereas the reduced-fat spread has more salt but is considerably lower in fat and calories. If these are foods that you use frequently, you would be much better off choosing the reduced-fat spread, as it could be used as part of a generally lower-calorie diet, which would help you lose weight and therefore reduce your blood pressure. If you chose the unsalted butter, it could only help reduce your blood pressure by a minute amount, but the cause of the high blood pressure (the excess body weight) would still remain.

Some foods are particularly high in salt, and so should be used sparingly. Sauces, such as those made with stock cubes, gravy granules, Bovril, and soy sauce, have a very high salt content. Other very salty foods include Marmite, cheese, pickles, and cured meats and fish. Other products such as tinned baked beans and ready meals vary in salt content from one brand to the next, and so it is best to check the nutrition information box on the packets to compare brands.

Alcohol

Alcohol has several effects that can hinder someone's ability to lose weight and feel healthy. Alcohol intake is measured in units, with one unit being equivalent to 1/2 pint of ordinary lager, a 125 ml glass of wine, or one pub measure of spirits. Note that premium lager contains 3 units of alcohol per pint and that wine is rarely sold in glasses as small as 125 ml, so it is very easy to drink far more than you realize.

1. Government recommendations advise women not to have more than 2–3 units of alcohol in any one day. Everyone should have at least 2 days per week on which they drink no alcohol at all. If a woman drinks more than 4 units in one day, this is classed as binge-drinking. These recommendations were drawn up to avoid complications of higher alcohol intakes, such as liver damage and certain cancers. It is worth bearing in mind that serving sizes of some alcoholic drinks have increased in recent years, so a large (250 ml) glass of wine actually provides 3 units of alcohol. As well as the long-term complications of excessive alcohol intake, in the short term it is responsible for a large number of accidents. Alcohol may also cause episodes of aggressive behaviour, which interestingly appear to be quite commonly reported by the women that attend our PCOS clinic.

2. Alcohol itself and alcoholic drinks contain a large number of calories, and so can be responsible for someone inadvertently taking in far more calories than they intend to. The table in Appendix 5 shows the calorie content of some common alcoholic drinks.

3. Alcohol stimulates the appetite, and so can cause people to eat more after they have been drinking than they would had they not been drinkng.

4. Alcohol increases the body's tendency to store fat, and so can make it harder to burn it off.

5. Taking in a large volume of alcohol causes people to lose control and be far less conscious of the food they should be eating and the exercise they should be doing.

See the case study below to see how large alcohol intakes may hinder your efforts to lose weight.

Patient's perspective

Helen has PCOS and has been losing weight at a rate of 1 lb per week for the last 5 weeks. She has done this by walking for 30 minutes every morning and restricting her food intake through keeping a food diary and preparing lower-calorie meals and snacks. She has been aiming to eat 1800 calories each day and is pleased with her progress so far. Today is Helen's 21st birthday. She goes for her 30 minute walk, feeling very positive. She has her usual breakfast, lunch, and between-meal fruit, and she feels even more positive when, at dinner with friends, she chooses a low-fat meal at the restaurant—she has definitely kept within her 1800 kcal. Then, however, the group goes to a bar after the meal and then on to a club. Whether she realizes it or not, by the end of the night Helen has drunk:

- 2 pints of premium lager (235 calories each)
- 4 alcopops (250 calories each)
- 3 shots of Sambuca (about 90 calories each).

When her friends drag her to the fast food shop on the way home and she smells the food, she orders a box of four pieces of fried chicken and chips (over 1100 calories), which she has completely devoured by the time she gets home. The following morning she does not feel like getting out of bed, so misses her morning walk and cooks her friends a fry-up instead.

Whereas Helen found that she could manage to stick to 1800 calories on a normal day, the night out drinking meant that she took in at least 4600 calories in just one day.

In this example, it is clear to see how it can be difficult to lose weight if you regularly drink alcohol to excess. Most people will drink too much at some point, but if you drink to excess every weekend then you may have to think about making alterations to your social life if you are serious about losing weight.

For more information about alcohol see www.nhsdirect.nhs.uk

Healthy eating—a summary

In summary, for most people, eating a healthier diet involves doing the following.

- Allow time to eat something for breakfast, lunch, and dinner everyday.
- Base meals on starchy foods (see Chapter 18 for which types are best for women with PCOS). These should account for about one-third of the food you eat.
- Consume at least five portions of a variety of fruit and vegetables every day. These should also account for about one-third of the food you eat.
- Decrease your intake of fatty and sugary foods and drinks. Eat foods containing fat, and foods and drinks containing sugar, sparingly.
- Enjoy a variety of different foods from each food group.
- Fluid is very important and may help to reduce your appetite. Drink a minimum of 1.2 litres of non-alcoholic fluids when the weather is cool and more when it is hotter, and make sure you are choosing low-calorie varieties.

I am really going to struggle with this. I don't like fruit or vegetables at all.

As the balanced diet model (Fig. 14.1) is the gold standard, it is something that we should be aiming towards. For example, if you currently eat only one portion of fruit or vegetable a day, setting yourself a goal to eat two portions per day would help you on your way to achieving this standard—do not feel you have to change everything all at once. Likewise, although it would be great to achieve this balance at every meal on every day, this is not essential provided that the balance is achieved over the course of a week or so. Remember that the proportion of foods shown includes snacks as well as meals.

For more information about healthy eating see the Foods Standards Agency website www.eatwell.gov.uk, and for more information about losing weight visit the British Dietetic Association's website www.bdaweightwise.com

However, just because someone eats very healthily, it does not necessarily mean that they will lose weight. Their 'healthy' diet may still provide the same number of calories as they are burning off. The next chapter will explain the facts about losing weight.

15

The physics of weight loss

 Key points

- You will only lose fat if you eat fewer calories than you are using up.
- The heavier someone is, the more calories they use up. Women with PCOS use almost the same number of calories as women of the same weight who do not have PCOS.
- One pound of fat stores 3,500 calories, so you will lose one pound of fat only as a result of eating 3,500 calories less than you have expended.

Myths about PCOS and weight loss

The following explanations are often given by women with PCOS for the difficulties they have with their weight.

- It's my hormones.
- I've got a slow metabolism.
- It's my glands.
- My whole family are overweight so it must be in my genes.
- I can't lose weight because I'm unable to exercise.

Before we explain any more about diet and weight loss, it is very important that you take on board the following piece of information.

Women with PCOS burn off almost the same number of calories as women without PCOS.

Imagine you have an identical twin sister, who is the same weight and height as you and who does the same level of activity as you everyday. She is identical to you in every way except that she does **not** have PCOS. What you would find is that, if you both ate exactly the same number of calories as each other every day for a year, if your twin sister's weight remained the same, yours would increase by 4 lb in that year. Therefore women with PCOS have a very slightly slower metabolism than their non-PCOS counterparts. An accumulation of 4 lb of fat in a year equates to an excess of only 38 calories per day, less than two teaspoons of sugar.

When I ask women in clinic how quickly they have gained weight, they usually respond by saying something like:

> about 2 stone in 8 months

or

> four stone since my son was born a year ago.

This level of weight gain cannot be explained merely by the slightly slower metabolism of women with PCOS. It is almost entirely due to the fact that women with PCOS have a tendency to eat more than women without PCOS. This is the main reason that PCOS makes it hard for you to control your weight—your high insulin level makes you hungrier and crave food more than a woman without PCOS, so you take in more calories than a woman without PCOS does. (For more information about the role of insulin in PCOS, see page 14.)

As I mentioned earlier, most women have tried every diet in existence by the time they come to see us in the PCOS clinic. Different commercial diets seem to produce varying degrees of success for different women, with most women reporting good weight loss on all diets. The main problems appeared to be either that they could not keep the weight off or that they did not think they had lost enough weight. The following facts may help to explain what makes diets work.

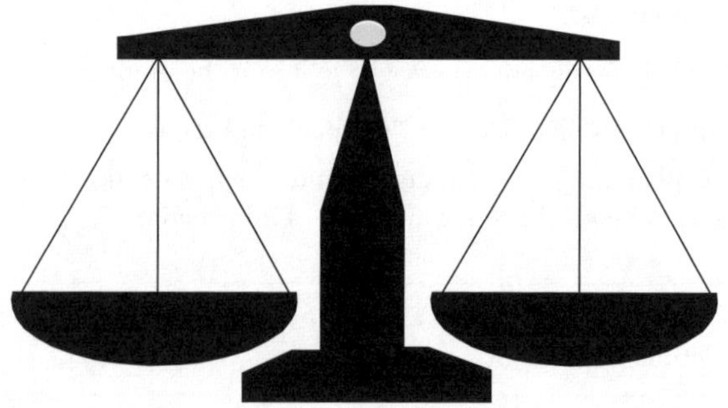

- If any diet causes you to restrict your food intake to the point where you are eating fewer calories than you are burning off, you will lose weight. If you eat more calories than you are burning off, you will gain weight.
- One pound of body fat stores 3500 calories—that's the same number of calories that you would find in 14 Mars bars!
  - That means to lose 1 lb of fat you must burn off 3500 calories more than you have eaten. This equates to you needing to eat 500 calories every day less than you are burning off to lose 1 lb of fat per week.
  - It also means that, in order for you to gain 1 lb of fat, you must eat 3500 calories more than you have burnt off. Simple!

What are calories?

A calorie is a measurement of energy. One thousand calories equals one kilocalorie (kcal). However, when talking about foods, we tend to use the word 'calorie' to mean 'kilocalorie'. In this book, every time the word 'calorie' is used, it is actually referring to 'kilocalorie'—everyone is familiar with the word 'calorie' so it is easier to understand! The energy we use up is measured in calories and, likewise, the amount of energy a food provides is measured in calories.

Energy expenditure

On average, 75 per cent of the calories we burn are used just to keep us alive. Our hearts use energy to pump blood around our bodies. Our nervous system uses energy to carry nerve impulses around our bodies. We also use up energy in maintaining our body temperature. Our bodies use up energy during the digestion of food. Then there's the energy we use up moving our bodies—the more we move, the more calories we use up. See Appendix 3 for details of the amount of energy used up during different forms of activity.

So, it is possible to lose weight even if you cannot do much exercise—it just means you have to restrict your calorie intake a bit further.

Muscle tissue uses up more calories than fat tissue. Therefore, preventing loss of muscle mass whilst you are losing fat can help prevent your metabolic rate decreasing as you lose weight. For this reason, as well as others, people who are active find it much easier to lose weight and keep it off.

Contrary to popular belief, the heavier you are the more calories you burn. Imagine you are 10 stone. If you had to go everywhere with a rucksack weighing 5 stone on your back, you would feel as if every task required a lot more effort. This is how it feels all the time for someone who weighs 15 stone.

Chapter 21 explains how you can work out the number of calories you burn off each day. The equations are produced by experts in weight management. (NB: Most yo-yo dieters think that these equations are for 'normal' people and that they burn off fewer calories than 'normal' people do. However, this is not the case—remember having PCOS only reduces your metabolic rate by around 38 calories per day!)

Work out your own energy expenditure—you might be surprised at how much you are burning off.

Energy input

Imagine you set fire to a pea. The pea would burn for a very short time before the flame disappeared and you were left with a pile of ash. Now imagine you set fire to a peanut. Although it is the same size as the pea, the peanut would burn for 12 times as long as the pea because it contains 12 times as much energy than the pea. A pea contains 2 calories while a peanut contains 24 calories. Therefore, eating 12 peas would provide you with the same number of calories as eating one peanut.

The number of calories a food or drink contains depends on the composition of the food or drink, or how much of it is made up of carbohydrate, protein, fat, and alcohol, and what proportion of it is made up of water. Table 15.1 shows the number of calories contributed by each of these nutrients. A pea is made up of mostly water with a little carbohydrate and protein, whereas a peanut is made up of mostly fat with some protein and carbohydrate, so this explains why a peanut contains far more calories than a pea. As you can see, fat contains more calories than any other nutrient, so an easy way to reduce your calorie intake is to reduce the amount of fat in your diet.

It is important to note that all types of fat have the same calorie content. Although we know that mono-unsaturated fats, such as olive oil and rapeseed oil, are the healthiest for our hearts, they are no less fattening than saturated fats, as their calorie content per gram is the same.

Table 15.1 Energy density of nutrients

Nutrient	Calories per gram
Water	0
Carbohydrate	3.75
Protein	4
Alcohol	7
Fat	9

PCOS, fats, and your heart

As a woman with PCOS, you have approximately seven times the risk of having a heart attack as a woman without PCOS. This risk rises the more overweight you are and rises dramatically if you also smoke.

We all have cholesterol in our blood. It is a type of fat which is bound to protein so that it can be carried around in the bloodstream. There are two main types of cholesterol—LDL-cholesterol and HDL-cholesterol. LDL-cholesterol is sometimes referred to as 'bad cholesterol', as it is carried from the liver into the bloodstream, where it can cause the arteries to narrow and harden. Having a raised level of LDL-cholesterol is associated with a higher risk of heart disease and stroke.

HDL-cholesterol is sometimes called 'good cholesterol', because it is carried from the blood back to the liver to be removed from the body, so it helps prevent the arteries becoming narrowed and blocked. Therefore, a higher level of HDL-cholesterol is associated with a lower risk of heart disease and stroke.

The levels of these two types of cholesterol are affected by the types of fat in our diets as well as by other factors such as insulin levels, activity, alcohol intake, genetics, and smoking. Table 15.2 shows how the different types of fat in the diet can affect your cholesterol.

Table 15.2 Effect of dietary fats on cholesterol levels

Fat	Found in	Effect on:	
		LDL	HDL
Saturates	Dairy or meat products Lard, palm oil, pastries, manufactured cakes/biscuits	↑	↑
Mono-unsaturates	Olive oil and spreads Rapeseed oil and spreads Nuts, peanut oil	↓	–
Poly-unsaturates	Sunflower oil and spreads Corn oil	↓	↓

As you can see, the mono-unsaturated fats are the ones which are best for your cholesterol levels, as they reduce the total cholesterol level without affecting the healthy HDL-cholesterol level.

The other type of fat that is often talked about is omega-3. This is a type of poly-unsaturated fat which is found in oily fish and in linseeds. It does not have much effect on your actual cholesterol level but is extremely good for your heart, as it helps prevent your blood becoming sticky and forming clots. When arteries are narrowed due to a build-up of plaque made from LDL-cholesterol, there is less room for the blood to pass through. If the blood is also quite sticky and likely to clot, there is a serious risk that a clot will completely block the already narrowed artery. When the blood cannot get through to the heart for a few seconds, part of the heart tissue will die as it receives no oxygen. This is what happens during a heart attack. A similar situation may occur in the brain and, when brain tissue is starved of oxygen, it causes a stroke. If you regularly take in omega-3 fats by eating oily fish, you will reduce the risk of a clot forming in your bloodstream and therefore reduce the risk of having a heart attack or stroke, irrespective of your cholesterol levels.

If you are not planning on having any children in the future, you can eat oily fish up to four times a week. The amount recommended for prevention of cardiovascular disease is 2–3 portions per week. However, due to safety concerns over toxins that may accumulate in oily fish, it is recommended that women of childbearing age do not consume more than two portions per week. For more information about your heart health, visit www.bhf.org.uk.

Have a look at the following two days' food intakes to see how variable calorie intakes can be.

Table 15.3 Comparison of two days' energy intakes

Day one	Day two
Two thick slices of toast with butter and jam at dining table	One thick slice of toast with olive spread and half tin baked beans at dining table
Can of Coke from machine at work, sipped at the desk	Apple at desk and can of diet Coke
Tuna mayonnaise baguette and packet of crisps in work canteen	Healthy option tuna sandwich and packet of Lite crisps eaten in work canteen
Two slices of toast with butter after work, eaten in the kitchen	Banana brought from home, eaten on way home from work
Chicken Kiev with oven chips and peas; pot of chocolate mousse, eaten on the sofa	Skinless chicken breast baked with garlic, oven chips, and peas; pot of 'light' chocolate mousse
Two packets of crisps whilst watching TV	Two gingernuts whilst watching TV
Four cups of tea throughout the day, each with semi-skimmed milk and two sugars	Four cups of tea throughout the day, each with semi-skimmed milk and one sweetener
Total calories = 3150	Total calories = 1499

The average woman burns off around 2000 calories per day. If she ate everyday with an excess of 1150 calories like day one in the example, she could actually gain eight and a half stone in a year. If she ate every day leaving a deficit of 500 calories, like day two in the example, she could lose 1 lb per week, or three and three-quarter stone in a year.

Still haven't lost weight? Interpreting weight changes

You are probably familiar with the situation whereby you weigh yourself on Friday morning, having been 'good' all week, and then you go out for a meal and a few glasses of wine on Friday night, only to weigh yourself on Saturday morning and discover that you've gained 3 lb. At this point you will probably panic, feel like all your hard work during the week was for nothing, and feel terribly guilty about the curry. Well fear not. Remember that to gain 1 lb of fat you must eat 3500 calories more than you have burnt off. Therefore, to have gained 3 lb of fat in one day, you would have had to have eaten 10 500 calories more than you had burnt off in that day.

The point is, it would be almost impossible to gain 3 lb of fat from just one meal, even if it were quite a high-calorie meal. The most likely explanations for this sudden increase in weight are as follows.

- When eating out, we tend to eat foods that are higher in salt than we would have eaten at home whilst eating a healthy diet. Our bodies have to keep the concentration of salt steady and therefore, when we take in more salt, we require more water to dilute this extra salt. Therefore, we tend to put on weight temporarily when we eat salty foods, but it is just extra fluid, not fat.
- In being 'good' all week you were eating fewer calories than you were burning off, so your body will have used up some of its carbohydrate stores before it went on to burn off fat. When we go out for a curry, we are likely to eat a great deal of carbohydrate—naan bread, rice, Bombay potatoes, and poppadums. This sudden increase in carbohydrate intake can cause temporary weight gain, as explained in the box below.

It is important to remember that you should be aiming to lose fat and not just weight. If you know you have taken in fewer calories than you have been burning off, you will have lost some fat even if your weight hasn't changed. As fat stores take a long time to increase or decrease, it is best to weigh yourself no more than once a week.

Carbohydrate stores

We can store approximately 1 lb of carbohydrate in our muscles and liver.

Our bodies store carbohydrate as glycogen—it's the animal equivalent of a plant storing starch.

This glycogen is used up when our food intake does not meet our bodies' requirement for energy.

In its stored form, each gram of glycogen is attached to 3–4 g of water.

Therefore, each time we use up a gram of glycogen, we get rid of an additional 3–4 g of water, and so using up the full pound of glycogen (almost 2000 calories worth) causes us to lose 4 or 5 lbs in total weight. This rapid loss of 4 or 5 lbs of carbohydrate and water is often demonstrated by people who are just starting to follow a low-carbohydrate diet.

Once we have used up our carbohydrate stores, we can replace them—and the additional water—quickly by eating a high-carbohydrate meal, causing us rapidly to regain the 4 lb of body weight, but not body fat.

16

Physical activity and weight management

 Key points

- Research has shown that individuals who are successful at losing weight and maintaining weight loss are likely to exercise for about an hour a day.
- Exercise helps weight loss by increasing energy expenditure, increasing insulin sensitivity, and enhancing metabolism.
- It is important that you develop an exercise programme that you find enjoyable and can fit into your busy life otherwise you will be unlikely to continue with it.

Exercise is any physical activity you do, from walking up the stairs to cleaning the house. It does not necessarily mean going to the gym. It is thought that most people today do not get enough exercise. There are fewer of us doing manual jobs and we are increasingly reliant on the car for transport. In the UK, both walking and cycling have declined by 25 per cent. Energy-saving devices such as washing machines, dishwashers and remote controls, in addition to the availability of home entertainment and computers, have also contributed to less active lifestyles. It is estimated that our energy expenditure may have reduced by as much as 30 per cent over the past three decades. Studies have shown a close link between being sedentary and being overweight.

Research has shown that the best way to lose weight successfully and keep the weight off over the long term is by a combination of making changes to your diet and increasing your levels of physical activity. By exercising, you will also feel better and have more energy, which will help you cope with the dietary changes. The National Weight Control Registry is a US database which provides information about the strategies used by over 4000 people who have lost more than 30 lb and kept it off for at least a year. It revealed that individuals

Table 16.1 Benefits of physical activity

Burns calories and may boost metabolism
Helps minimize weight gain
Protects against osteoporosis
Helps to protect against high blood pressure and reduce the risk of heart disease
Helps to lower cholesterol and reduce the risk of developing diabetes
May reduce the risk of developing colon and breast cancer
Helps improve self-image and mood
Helps to reduce stress
Improves muscle strength
Improves flexibility

who were successful at maintaining weight loss were likely to exercise for about an hour a day. Research has also shown that adults who are physically active have a 30 per cent reduced risk of premature death compared with those who live sedentary lives, and are half as likely to develop diseases such as diabetes, certain cancers, and heart disease (Table 16.1).

How exercise helps weight loss

Energy expenditure

You will burn calories by moving body weight, so any movement built into your daily routine will result in an increase in energy expenditure. If you use up more calories than you consume you will lose weight. Heavier people have the advantage that they use more energy for the same task than a lighter person because they have more weight to carry. The intensity of the activity determines how many calories are used up—the harder the work, the more calories burned and the more fat lost.

The table in Appendix 3 gives examples of the amount of calories burned during different activities at different body weights.

Insulin sensitivity

Remember that insulin is the hormone that is responsible for the uptake of glucose (sugar) by the cells of the body to be used as energy. If you are insulin resistant, then insulin is not working as efficiently as it should and so your pancreas has to produce higher than normal amounts of insulin to compensate. This high level of insulin encourages the conversion of glucose to fat rather than being used up as energy, leaves you feeling tired and hungry, and gives you sugar cravings. Numerous trials have shown that regular exercise increases the body's responsiveness to insulin, thereby increasing glucose uptake by the muscle cells and reducing blood insulin levels. A recent study in women with PCOS has confirmed that insulin levels can be reduced by moderate exercise even if there is no associated weight loss. However, trials have also shown that insulin levels are further reduced by losing weight as the less body fat there is, the better the insulin sensitivity.

Getting started

Increasing your physical activity does not have to mean going to the gym. Review how much physical activity you do in a day and think about ways to increase it. Small changes in routine can increase your energy expenditure over the week and contribute to weight management. For example:

- Take the stairs instead of using the lift or escalator
- Handwash your car
- Do the housework at a fast pace
- Do not use remote control for your television or music system—get out of your chair to change channels, CDs, etc., instead
- Walk the dog regularly
- Walk to the station instead of driving.
- Park the car a distance from work or the shops and walk the rest of the way.

Walking is one of the best forms of physical activity. It is cheap, you do not need any special equipment, and it is unlikely to injure you. Try to walk briskly so that you are slightly out of breath to gain maximum benefit. Buy a pedometer (it clips on your belt and measures how many steps you take) and gradually increase the number of steps you take each day by 250–500 steps or whatever you feel comfortable with. The British Heart Foundation suggests a target of 10 000 steps per day to be healthy, and if you want to lose weight then you should gradually increase this to 15 000 steps a day.

It is important that you develop an exercise programme that you find enjoyable and can fit into your busy life otherwise you will be unlikely to continue

Table 16.2 Your physical activity goals

	To keep fit	To lose weight and minimize weight regain
Frequency	5 times a week	Daily
Intensity	At least moderate intensity, enough to make you out of breath and sweaty	At least moderate intensity, enough to make you out of breath and sweaty
Types	Cardiovascular activities you enjoy	Activities you enjoy—mainly cardiovascular but include resistance training twice a week
Time	30 minutes a day	60 minutes a day. How long you are active will determine how many calories you burn each day

with it. Aim to increase the amount of physical activity gradually to a frequency of at least 30 minutes a day (try 3 × 10 minute bursts if that is easier for you). If you are not used to exercise, start off slowly for a short time, say 10–15 minutes. Start off with any activity a couple of times a week. After 2–3 weeks increase the number of times per week but keep the length of time the same. After another couple of weeks, increase the time that you do your activity by a few minutes. Always listen to your body—if you feel dizzy or nauseous, or develop pain, then you must stop. If you have a medical condition such as high blood pressure, heart disease, or asthma then you should see your doctor first so that he/she can advise you on what is the best form of exercise for you. You should also speak to your doctor if you are pregnant.

Once you have got yourself into the habit of doing 30 minutes of exercise five times a week, try to increase this gradually if possible over a course of a few weeks to 60 minutes (can be divided into 10–15 minute sessions) daily (Table 16.2).

Types of exercise

There are two types of exercise, both of which burn calories.

Aerobic or cardiovascular exercise

This causes you to breathe harder and makes your heart work harder to pump blood around the body as evidenced by an increase in your heart rate. Examples are walking, swimming, cycling, and tennis. Performed on a regular basis, it improves the health of your heart and lungs in addition to burning body fat. You will need to exercise hard enough to increase your heart rate and breathing. When you first start to exercise you should aim for your heart rate to reach 60 per cent of your maximum heart rate. This is your 'target heart rate'. As your fitness improves you can exercise harder and increase your target heart rate to 80 per cent of your maximum heart rate.

Your maximum heart rate is worked out as: 220 – your age
Target heart rate = maximum heart rate × 0.6 or 0.8

Weight or resistance training

This form of exercise builds muscle strength and increases your muscle mass. The more muscle you have the higher your metabolism will be, which means that you will burn more calories even when you are not exercising. Muscle needs up to 25 times as many calories to maintain as an equivalent weight of fat. Men have a higher metabolic rate than women because they have more muscle mass. Resistance training also helps reduce the risk of osteoporosis, or brittle bones. Examples of resistance training include lifting weights, squats, and push ups. Ideally, you should aim to do resistance exercises twice a week with at least 1 day of rest between the two sessions to allow your muscles to recover. If you have not done resistance training before, then you may benefit from a personal trainer or gym instructor who can show you how to do the exercises properly and can help you design an individualized programme so that you achieve your goals safely.

It is worth bearing in mind that any physical activity (but particularly resistance training) may result in some increase in muscle mass, especially if it follows a period of relative inactivity. This increase in muscle mass can help you to burn off more calories at rest and it improves your insulin sensitivity. However, it may cause those women who are trying to lose weight to feel as though they are not achieving their weight loss targets. In this case it is particularly important that you keep some other measure of success as well as measuring your weight. If you can see centimetres coming off your waist or your trousers becoming looser, then this demonstrates that you are reducing your fat stores, regardless of the fact that your weight may not have changed.

Tips to help keep you more active

- Get a good pair of trainers and a sports bra.
- Always warm up and stretch for 5–10 minutes before exercising and cool down and stretch for a similar time after exercising. This is important to avoid muscle injuries.

- Drink plenty of water before, during, and after exercise. Initial weight loss is largely due to loss of water so you need to drink enough water in order to avoid dehydration. Furthermore, if you are dehydrated, you tend not to burn off fat efficiently.

- Set aside regular time to exercise—book it in your diary. You will then be less likely to make other arrangements instead. If you stick to the same time every day or week then your exercise will become part of your routine.

- Choose something you like doing and vary what you do so you do not get bored, for example walk one day, cycle the next day, and swim another day.

- Try and exercise with a friend. This will make it more fun and you will motivate, encourage, and support each other.

- Take up a hobby that involves being active, e.g. swimming, dancing, skating, gardening.

- Start slowly and gradually increase the length of time spent being active.

- Set yourself achievable and realistic weekly and monthly goals, and then track your progress. Be specific—how many steps do you intend to walk in a week? How many pounds do you aim to lose in a month? Reward yourself when you achieve your goals, for example a new top or a manicure. If there is a setback and you do not achieve your goal immediately, then do not give up but just reset the goal, make sure it is realistic, and try again. If you set yourself unrealistic goals, for example losing 4 stone in 4 months, you will become de-motivated and will be more likely to give up. Remember that you're in this for the long haul. Anything you undertake too intensely may quickly become too onerous, and you'll be more likely to give it up.

- Keep an exercise diary to monitor your progress and help you focus on achieving your goals.

- Find time for exercise—get up an hour early, walk in your lunch break, use an exercise bike while watching television. Remember you do not have to do 30 minutes of activity all at once—you can divide your physical activity into three 10 minute sessions or two 15 minute sessions if that is easier to fit into your day.

- Don't get discouraged—it may seem a struggle at first but it does become easier and more enjoyable with time.

17

Preparing to lose weight

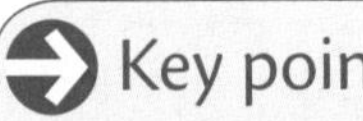

Key points

- Research has shown that people who write down everything they eat and drink, as they eat it, are more successful at losing weight.
- Keeping a food and activity diary can help you identify problems with your current lifestyle, which can then be overcome by setting yourself goals.
- Your goals should be specific, measurable, achievable and realistic. Success breeds success, so avoid setting goals which you are unlikely to achieve.

If you fail to prepare, prepare to fail…

If you have read Chapters 13–16 of this book then you have already completed the first stage in planning to lose weight. If you have got this far, then you will have established that you have the motivation to make changes to your lifestyle and behaviour, and you should have realistic expectations of losing weight.

Changing well-established habits is a difficult thing to do and takes careful planning and consideration. In the same way that someone would find it very difficult to give up smoking if they continued to buy cigarettes from the supermarket each week, you will find it difficult to burn off more calories than you are consuming unless you make some changes to your behaviour.

Self-monitoring

People who regularly monitor their weight and food intake are much more likely to succeed at losing weight and keeping it off. Studies have consistently shown that people who are overweight underestimate their food and calorie intake by as much as 50 per cent. Likewise, people who are underweight over-report what they are eating by 50 per cent. This happens, not because these people are intentionally lying, but because they have developed a very skewed idea of what they are actually eating.

Everyone who is overweight knows someone who is skinny but appears to eat 'whatever they like'. This may be the case, but the fact is that the skinny friend is only skinny because she eats fewer calories than her overweight counterpart. Remember that the heavier you are the more calories you use up, so the skinny person must eat very few calories in order to maintain her low weight. Slim women may purposely eat high-fat foods in public and they may even enjoy the comments they receive from their envious overweight friends.

Aren't you lucky being able to eat whatever you like—I just have to look at a piece of cake ...!

However, it is the overweight women (who usually avoid eating high-calorie foods in public) who end up eating more calories without realizing it. We often remember only the meals we have sat down to eat, whilst we forget the foods we eat outside of mealtimes.

- The odd slice of ham or piece of cheese whilst standing at the fridge
- The biscuit eaten in the kitchen whilst we are making a cup of tea
- The ingredients munched whilst we prepare a meal
- The additional slice-worth of cake we eat whilst 'tidying up' the crumbs on the side of the slice we've just eaten
- The nibbling of children's left-overs
- The wine and meals or snacks eaten when we go out
- The sweets eaten in the car after stopping for petrol.

Every single morsel of food we eat provides us with calories, and it is usually these additional uncontrolled calories that make the difference between losing weight and not losing weight. Making a written note of everything you eat draws your attention to the food you're eating and therefore you are likely to eat considerably less whilst you keep writing it down. It can also help to highlight problems—for example it may be that you eat too many biscuits mid-morning on the days that you skip breakfast. Studies have consistently shown that people who write down everything they eat are more successful at losing weight than people who don't keep a food diary.

You are most likely to be successful at losing weight if you write down everything you eat as you eat it. See the following two patients' stories.

Patients' perspectives

Faye, 34 years

As part of her weight loss plan, Faye is keeping a food diary, but she has left it in the kitchen. She has just sat down on the sofa to watch her favourite television programme and she's brought a full packet of chocolate digestive biscuits in with her from the kitchen to save herself getting up in the middle of the programme. Three hours later she is still watching television and the entire contents of the biscuit packet appear to have vanished. When she returns to the kitchen, she writes in her food diary 'About 20 chocolate digestive biscuits' and realizes with dismay that, as each biscuit contains 80 calories, she's just eaten about 1600 calories as a snack.

Jo, 27 years

As part of her weight loss plan, Jo is keeping a food diary—a pocket-sized book, which she carries with her everywhere. She has just sat down on the sofa to watch her favourite television programme and she's brought a full packet of chocolate digestive biscuits in with her from the kitchen to save herself getting up in the middle of the programme. She eats one biscuit and writes down '1 chocolate digestive' in her diary. She then eats another biscuit and writes '1 chocolate digestive' in her diary. By the time she has written '1 chocolate digestive' four times, she considers how many she has eaten and why she is eating them. She is aware that four biscuits amounts to 320 calories. After thinking about why she is eating them she considers whether there is, in fact, any reason why she should continue eating them. She decides that she has enjoyed those four biscuits and does not need any more, so she gets up and puts them back in the kitchen.

As you can see from these examples, writing down everything you eat at the time of eating it can help you to become much more aware of what you are eating and why you are eating it. By doing this, monitoring your own food intake can actually help you to eat considerably fewer calories.

A food and activity diary is therefore an essential item to have if you are serious about losing weight. It can help you identify problems with your eating pattern, times when you are most likely to take in excess calories, and particular triggers to overeating. Your diary is for you, and no one else, to see, so be as accurate and honest with yourself as possible.

Your food and activity diary should be small enough that you can always carry it with you. It should contain the following columns.

1. When? The times you are eating can help you identify problems with your meal pattern. Do you skip breakfast and end up accepting biscuits, when offered them mid-morning, because you are hungry?

2. Where? Do you frequently eat out? Do you sit down at a table to eat and therefore feel like you have had a proper meal? Or do you eat whilst standing at the fridge? Do you eat your dinner on the sofa in front of the TV or do you actually pay attention to your food whilst you are eating it?

3. What and how much? If you are trying to eat a certain number of calories each day you should be as accurate as you can in this column. This way you will not under- or overestimate your portion sizes and therefore your energy intake. If you are the type of person who grazes throughout the day, the portion sizes are not so important—it is more useful to identify why your eating pattern is like this so that you can do something about it.

4. Thoughts/feelings/triggers. Do you eat more when you are stressed or tired? When the children have gone to bed? When your partner has gone out? When your friend or partner brings you treats? How do you feel after you have eaten it? Filling in this column can help you to identify what is making you eat in the way you do and, from this, you can plan how you will behave next time you are in that situation. For example, the next time you become stressed, you could run a nice warm bath and paint your nails to make you feel relaxed and positive instead of eating chocolate and making yourself feel guilty and negative. Food diaries are the most useful way of drawing your attention to the times you eat when you are not actually hungry.

5. Activity. This can make a very significant contribution to the 'output' side of the energy balance equation. Write down all the activity you do and how long you spend on each activity. It will make you realize how well you are doing and give you more incentive to increase the amount of activity you do. If you have a pedometer, writing down the number of steps you take daily is a good idea. If you find being active difficult, you could write down the amount of time you spend being sedentary instead (include all time spent sitting still). You can then aim to reduce the amount of time you spend each day on sedentary activities.

Other considerations

Before you start your weight loss plan, consider the following six points:

1. **Do I have support from the people around me?**
   - Do you live with someone else? Do they encourage you or do they nag you? Do they bring home 'treats' which sabotage your efforts to lose weight?
   - Do your friends or colleagues keep offering you high-calorie foods?
     - ➤ Talk to the people around you. Explain how important losing weight is to you and that you would really appreciate their help rather than them making it more difficult for you. Remember that other people will often offer you high-calorie foods to make themselves feel less guilty about eating them. Partners often think they are being helpful by saying things like 'Should you really be eating that?', when in fact this approach is likely to make you want to eat it even more. So speak to them gently and let them know how they could be more encouraging rather than nagging.
2. **When am I going to buy food?**
   - Do you buy food for your household or is the shopping done by someone else?
   - Do you do the food shopping at a time when you are hungry?
     - ➤ If the food you are going to eat is bought by someone else then it is important that you talk to them about your plans, so that they can buy the foods that you want.
     - ➤ If you are responsible for the food shopping then you are in control. You will buy more food, and specifically more high-calorie foods, if you shop when you are hungry. So pick a time when you can do the food shopping straight after a meal.
3. **What food am I going to buy?**
   - Do you cruise the aisles of the supermarket, being tempted by the aromas and the 'special offers'?
     - ➤ Shopping lists are very useful tools. Having some idea of the meals you are going to eat during the week and writing down all the foods you will need for those meals means that you can go straight to the appropriate sections of the supermarket. By doing this you will avoid having to walk past the foods that you hadn't planned to buy.

- Doing your weekly supermarket shop on the Internet can also be helpful, as you can simply enter the foods you need to buy and are not tempted to impulse-buy the foods that you would normally see and smell in the supermarket.
- Be prepared: if you know that some days you are going to be too rushed to spend ages cooking, then plan for this by buying some quick healthy meals such as 'Healthy Option' ready meals or pre-prepared stir-fries. This way you will be less likely to end up ordering a take-away when you are short of time.

4. **How can I stop myself buying things that I know are a problem?**
   - Do you buy high-calorie meals, snacks, or drinks from vending machines or the cafeteria at work?
   - Do you pass a bakery or coffee shop on a journey that you make frequently?
   - Do you often buy snacks when you stop to fill your car with petrol?
     - You may be aware of times that are a particular problem for you. If, for example, you know you usually buy a chocolate bar from the machine at work, you could try leaving your cash at home, or bring enough cash for the bus only.
     - Have you thought about walking a different way so that you don't have to walk past the bakery? If so, you might find you increase your activity level at the same time as avoiding the pastries.
     - In the same way that you would try to go to the supermarket on a full stomach to avoid impulse-buying, you could try to be prepared and fill your car up with petrol after a meal when possible.

5. **How am I going to find the time for physical activity?**
   - Do you currently use the bus or car for short journeys?
   - Do you frequently use lifts or escalators?
   - How much time do you currently spend watching TV or on a home computer?
     - If you are worried about finding time to be more active, make sure that you make the best use of everyday activities such as walking and always taking the stairs instead of the lift.
     - It may be helpful for you to use a pedometer to find out how many steps you are walking at the moment. If you find you are not doing many, you may be more inclined to increase the number.

➤ If you still cannot see any way of increasing your activity levels, aim instead to reduce the amount of time you spend on sedentary activities such as watching television, reading, or using a computer. The less time you spend sitting down, the more active you will be without even realizing it, as you may be doing housework or gardening instead. Spending less time sitting down might help you to eat less too!

6. **How am I going to make it easy for myself to monitor my food intake and my weight?**
   - Have you prepared yourself a food and activity diary?
   - Is the diary of such a size that you can take it with you whenever you think you may eat something, including foods eaten outside the home?
     - ➤ It is useful to start keeping a food and activity diary even before you try to change your eating and activity habits. This way you will be able to identify the problems in your current behaviour, so that you can make the necessary changes to solve the problem.
     - ➤ It is also worth preparing a record of your weekly weights and occasional waist and hip measurements to track your progress. This might be included as part of your food diary or it might be a separate sheet; it doesn't matter as long as you can see how well you are doing.

Goal setting

As part of the preparation stage, you may start to think about what your goals are going to be. When setting yourself any kind of goal, it is important to consider whether your goals are SMART.

- S pecific
- M easurable
- A chievable
- R ealistic
- T ime-limited

For example, you may decide that you'd like to become more active. You would need to alter your goal in the following ways to ensure that it is SMART.

- Specific—I'm going to walk more and go to the gym.
- Measurable—I'm going to walk with a pedometer and aim for a certain number of steps each day and do the whole gym programme set for me by my fitness instructor when I go to the gym.

- Achievable—I'm going to see how many steps I'm walking at the moment and my goal will be to walk this far plus an extra 1000 steps each day. I'm going to do my programme at the gym three times a week.
- Realistic—My goal is to walk an extra 1000 steps per day on 5 days per week and to do my gym programme three times a week on a good week and at least once during a week when going to the gym will be difficult.
- Time-limited—I'm going to review my achievements in a month's time and consider increasing my goal if I can.

We can't emphasize enough the importance of being realistic and flexible when you are setting yourself goals. Imagine you set yourself a goal to do your whole gym programme 5 days per week. Now imagine that you had to work late on Monday, Tuesday, and Wednesday. By not going to the gym for 3 days you might end up thinking, 'Well, it's impossible for me to go to the gym five times this week, so I might as well not go at all. I'll start again next week'. You may then find yourself in the situation where you feel guilty for not going to the gym instead of feeling good about yourself when you do go. As with any kind of target setting, only set yourself a goal that will result in you feeling good about yourself. If your goal is likely to be unattainable, then the chances are that it will actually make you feel worse about yourself and reduce your confidence.

18

Polycystic ovary syndrome, carbohydrates, and the glycaemic index

 Key points

- Women with PCOS are usually insensitive to insulin, which results in an overproduction of insulin to compensate.
- Insulin in high levels causes hormonal imbalances which are responsible for all the symptoms of PCOS. Insulin also prevents the breakdown of fat, making weight loss more difficult.
- Choosing a diet based on foods with a lower glycaemic index can help reduce hunger and cravings, and may help reduce the amount of insulin produced.

Women with PCOS tend to fall into one of two groups: those who crave sweet foods (such as chocolate, cakes, sweets, crunchy nut cornflakes, etc.) and those who crave savoury foods (such as bread, pizza, mashed potato, etc.). All these women, regardless of which group they belong to, are actually craving the same thing—carbohydrates.

The reason women with PCOS crave carbohydrates is that their insulin does not work properly. Let us explain.

Digestion of carbohydrates

Carbohydrates in food exist as sugars and starch (Figure 18.1).

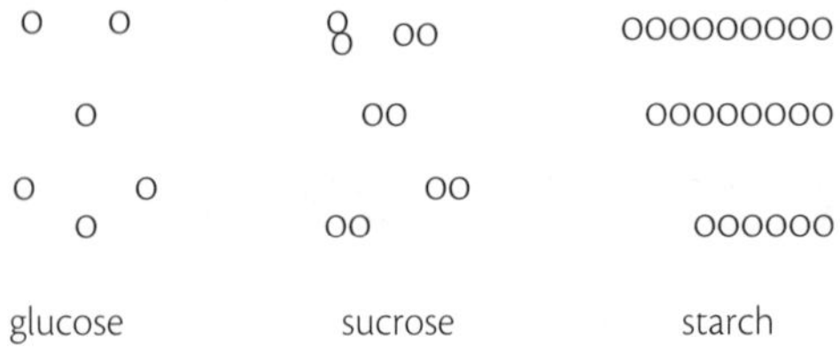

glucose sucrose starch

Figure 18.1 Structure of carbohydrates.

When we take in glucose, as an energy drink such as Lucozade or as dextrose tablets (dextrose is another name for glucose), the glucose is absorbed through the wall of our intestine immediately and passes straight into the blood, causing our blood glucose level to rise rapidly.

As you can see from Fig. 18.1, glucose is made up of just one unit. Along with glucose, there are other types of monosaccharides, or 'single sugars', including fructose, the main type of sugar found in fruit. Although fructose is absorbed quickly like glucose, it passes into the bloodstream as fructose and therefore does not cause the actual blood glucose level to rise very much at all.

Sucrose is the chemical name for the stuff we add to our tea and coffee, sprinkle on our cereal and strawberries, and mix into cakes and puddings. Whether it be caster or granulated, brown or white, demerara or muscovado, it is still sucrose. Sucrose is made up of one glucose unit and one fructose unit and, because it is made up of two sugar units, it is known as a disaccharide. Only the glucose unit in sucrose has the capacity to raise blood glucose levels rapidly, and so, gram for gram, sucrose increases the blood glucose less rapidly than glucose does.

Lactose is another disaccharide and is the sugar that occurs naturally in milk. It is responsible for making the 'Nutrition Information' panel on the side of a pot of diet yoghurt very confusing, as it appears that there is a great deal of sugar in the yoghurt, yet there is no added sugar on the list of ingredients. This sugar is lactose: a combination of glucose and another monosaccharide called galactose. Lactose takes some time to be broken down into its monosaccharide units, so does not cause our blood glucose levels to rise very quickly.

Starch is a type of polysaccharide ('many sugars') and consists of long chains of glucose units joined together. These starch molecules are too big to be absorbed through our intestine as they are, and so they need to be broken down into smaller pieces. For this reason, an organ in our digestive tract called the pancreas secretes juices into the intestine, which allow glucose units to be broken off, bit by bit, from the ends of the starch chains. In this way, starches

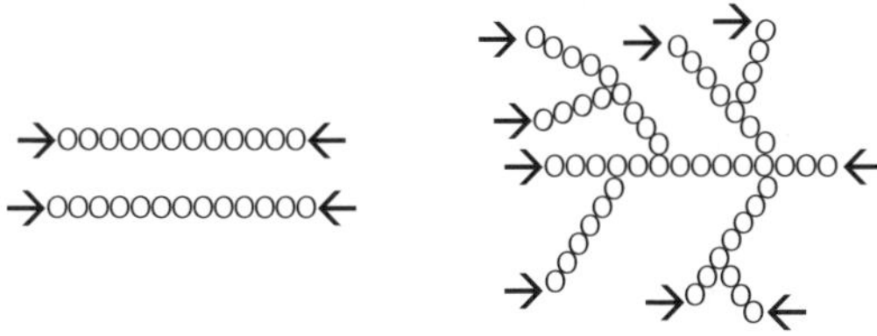

Figure 18.2 Straight-chain carbohydrates versus branched carbohydrates.

are digested into sugar, in order to make particles small enough to be absorbed through the wall of our intestine and into the blood.

Different types of starch are broken down into glucose at different rates, depending on how straight or branched the starch chains are, as the digestive juices can only remove glucose units from the ends of the chains.

For example, if you looked at jasmine rice through an extremely powerful microscope, you would find that the starch chains have lots of branches, allowing lots of glucose units to be broken off at once, as shown in Fig. 18.2. This is because jasmine rice contains more of a type of starch called amylopectin, which is branched. This branching allows more water to be held within the starch, making it even quicker to digest. Basmati rice, however, is made up more of amylase, the straighter-chained starch molecules, allowing fewer glucose units to be broken off at a time. Therefore, basmati rice is turned into glucose much more slowly than jasmine rice, causing a slower rise in the blood glucose level.

Carbohydrates, insulin, and appetite

Our bodies are programmed to keep our blood glucose level within a certain range (usually between 4 and 8 millimoles per litre of blood). Whenever we eat food, the carbohydrate in the food is absorbed into the blood and our blood glucose level begins to rise. Our bodies can detect this rise in blood glucose and we respond by secreting insulin into the blood from the pancreas; that is the same organ that previously squirted the digestive juice into the intestine to break down the starch.

Insulin is a hormone, or chemical messenger, that tells channels to open between our blood vessels and our muscle cells, in order to allow the glucose to pass from the bloodstream into the muscles, where it will be used to fuel their movement. In this way, insulin allows the glucose to come out of the bloodstream, preventing the blood glucose level from becoming too high. Nowadays, however, most of us are too inactive to keep using up the glucose in our muscles, so sometimes our muscles have no space to store any more glucose. When this situation occurs, the insulin causes channels to open from the blood vessels into the fat cells, so the glucose is able to enter the fat cells to be turned into fat for storage.

As explained in Chapter 2, most women with PCOS are insensitive to insulin, so have to secrete several times as much insulin as women without PCOS do, to prevent their blood glucose level becoming too high. The result is that women with PCOS have a high level of insulin circulating in their blood and this has several effects.

- High levels of insulin make your ovaries produce more testosterone, which may cause you to experience the symptoms of unwanted hair growth, menstrual irregularities, acne, and male-pattern baldness.
- Insulin opens channels to allow glucose from the blood to enter muscle and fat cells. These channels only allow the passage of glucose in one direction and that is from the blood into the cells for storage. Therefore, while there are high levels of insulin in your blood it is difficult to break down fat. High insulin levels also make you more likely to store excess fat around your middle, so women with PCOS are more likely to be 'apple' shaped rather than 'pear' shaped, making shopping for jeans a particularly onerous task.

Waist circumference in women

Increased risk of health problems

Over 80 cm (32 inches)

Very increased risk of health problems

Over 88 cm (35 inches)

Having high levels of insulin in your bloodstream may cause alterations in other factors known to increase your risk of heart disease and stroke. People who are insulin resistant are often found to have a high level of fat called triglyceride in their blood. High triglyceride levels are associated with a higher risk of cardiovascular disease and may also be responsible for a 'fatty liver'. In addition, if you are insulin resistant, you are likely to have a low level of HDL (good) cholesterol in your blood and possibly a raised level of LDL (bad) cholesterol. High insulin levels can also cause your blood pressure to rise. High triglycerides, low HDL-cholesterol, high LDL-cholesterol, and high blood pressure are all individual risk factors for heart disease and stroke, and they can all be improved by losing a modest amount of weight and reducing your insulin levels. The most important effect that insulin resistance has on women with PCOS, in terms of weight gain, is this:

- Insulin resistance can make you more hungry and may make you crave carbohydrate foods.

Imagine you are sitting down to your healthy evening meal of jacket potato with salad and just a tiny sprinkle of strong grated cheese to melt on the top, just as most slimming clubs might recommend. You feel very pleased with yourself for eating such a healthy meal, but it's almost inevitable that about an hour after eating your big baked potato, despite feeling that your stomach is full, you will begin to just fancy something else to eat ... possibly something a bit sweet .... Having looked around the house and found some chocolate, which you then promptly munch, you are left feeling guilty and nowhere near as pleased with yourself as you did after your 'healthy' dinner. Familiar story?

When the potato leaves your stomach and enters your intestine, it begins to be broken down into glucose. Baking potatoes contain a type of starch that is digested and absorbed very quickly, and so the glucose level in your blood rises rapidly, causing a large amount of insulin, as well as some stress hormones, to be released to bring your blood glucose level back down. Following a high GI meal, you may eventually begin to experience the familiar carbohydrate cravings, even though you are not necessarily hungry.

What is the glycaemic index?

The glycaemic index, or GI, was first described by Professor Jenkins and his colleagues in 1981 after they had noticed that different types of carbohydrates exerted different effects on people's blood glucose. Jenkins went on to develop a method of ranking foods according to the extent and speed at which they increase blood glucose levels.

In order to work out the GI of different foods, Jenkins and his colleagues took a group of fasting people and measured their blood glucose level constantly for 2 hours after they had consumed 50 g of glucose. The same group of people were allowed to fast again and were then given 50 g of carbohydrate from a test food and their blood glucose levels were measured in the same way as they were after the glucose. In this example, they were testing porridge, so they were given about 350 g of porridge to provide 50 g carbohydrate (Fig. 18.3).

As you can see from Fig. 18.3, the porridge caused a much slower rise in blood glucose levels than the glucose. In fact, as glucose does not need to be broken

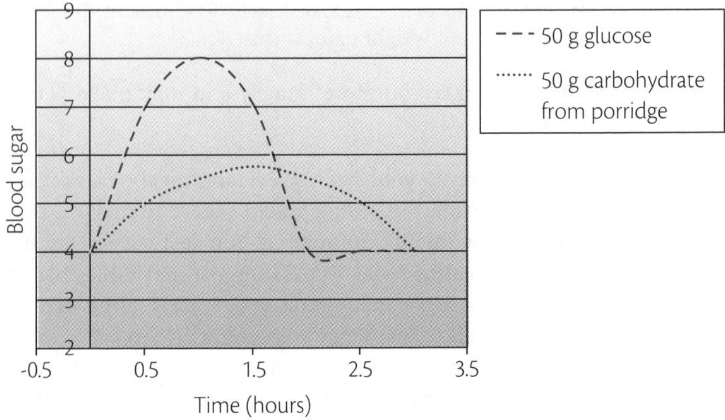

Figure 18.3 Glucose response to a high-GI food (glucose) and a low-GI food (porridge).

down into smaller units before it can be absorbed, it causes a very quick rise in blood glucose and therefore is usually used as the reference point. Glucose is given an arbitrary GI of 100, against which all other foods are compared. The area under the curve for all test foods is divided by the area under the curve for glucose to determine the GI, giving porridge a GI of around 52.

How can a low-GI diet help weight loss?

When you eat high-GI foods, your blood glucose rises rapidly and therefore a large surge of insulin is released into your bloodstream which rapidly removes this extra glucose from the blood. You are likely to crave some type of carbohydrate food shortly after eating a high-GI meal, even if you know you are not really hungry. By eating meals based on lower-GI starchy foods, you should feel satisfied for longer. In addition, you will help keep your insulin levels lower and therefore burn fat more easily.

In addition, in order to help keep your insulin levels down, it helps enormously if you avoid taking in any unnecessary carbohydrate in the form of drinks, as sugar in drinks is absorbed more rapidly, causing your insulin levels to peak every time you drink them. Sugary drinks also provide a large number of calories, which will not help you lose weight.

The table in Appendix 6 ranks some common carbohydrate foods according to whether they are high, medium, or low GI.

- The low-GI list consists of foods with a GI of 54 or less.
- The medium-GI list consists of foods with a GI from 55 to 69.
- The high-GI list consists of foods found to have a GI of 70 or above.

Therefore, in brief, your diet can be transformed into a lower-GI diet by swapping all sugary drinks for low-calorie alternatives and by choosing lower-GI varieties of breads, potatoes, rice, and pasta. For more information about GI, including a comprehensive list of the GI values of a vast number of foods, visit www.glycemicindex.com

It is important to realize that the GI of a food is not always a good indication of how healthy or how calorie dense the food is. For example, fructose, the sugar found in fruit, is absorbed differently from sucrose, or table sugar, and it doesn't cause the blood glucose level to rise quickly. However, it contains exactly the same number of calories, gram for gram, as sucrose. Using fructose in place of sucrose will not, therefore, help you to lose weight unless your appetite and subsequent food intake is reduced as a result of using a lower-GI sugar.

The presence of fat in a food actually slows down the rate at which the digested carbohydrates are absorbed, which explains why biscuits, chocolate, and cakes often have a lower GI than one might expect. These foods may have a low GI, but they are extremely high in calories and provide very few nutrients apart from fat and sugar. They should therefore still only be eaten as an occasional treat.

The presence of protein in a food or meal can also slow down the absorption of the carbohydrate, thereby lowering the GI of the food with which is it eaten. Pasta is usually made from durum wheat, which has a high protein content. This is one reason why the GI of pasta is so much lower than that of bread.

It is useful to bear in mind this GI-lowering effect of protein, as you can add protein to a high-GI food to make a lower-GI meal. For instance, adding baked beans or tuna, which are high in protein, to a jacket potato or wholemeal toast, which are high GI, will result in a medium-GI meal.

What about glycaemic load?

The glycaemic load (GL) is the name given to the product of the GI of a food and its carbohydrate content. It is a useful concept to consider, as it helps to give a clearer idea of how much the food will increase the blood glucose level. Let's look at two examples—watermelon versus Snickers bar. Watermelon has a GI of 76 (high) whereas the Snickers bar has a GI of 41 (low). The GI does not take into account the amount of carbohydrate in the foods, as all foods are tested using the amount required to provide 50 g of carbohydrate. Therefore, when the GI testing took place, the subjects would have been asked to consume enough watermelon to provide them with 50 g of carbohydrate—that's about 700 g of watermelon flesh. Likewise, when testing the GI of Snickers, subjects would have been asked to consume enough Snickers to provide them with 50 g of carbohydrate—that's about 90 g of Snickers. So although the watermelon has the high GI, you'd have to eat a whole watermelon at once to bring about that rise in blood glucose! Because people don't usually eat whole watermelons, the GL is more useful in this case than the GI.

The GL is calculated by multiplying the GI of the food by the number of grams of carbohydrate in a serving of that food and dividing the result by 100.

Watermelon contains 7 g of carbohydrate per 100 g serving so that this amount has a GL of 5. A Snickers bar contains 34 g of carbohydrate per 61 g bar and so has a GL of 14.

19

Alternative dietary approaches

Key points

- Different dietary approaches suit different people. Some women with PCOS seem to find it easier to eat fewer calories if they eat less carbohydrate, but the long-term safety of low carbohydrate diets remains controversial.
- Structured meal plans such as those which use balanced meal-replacement products may help people control their calorie intake.
- There is no evidence that any quick fix 'diet' will help people lose weight and keep it off. If a diet sounds too good to be true, it probably is.

Low-carbohydrate diets

Most people consume more than 200 g of carbohydrate daily as part of a normal balanced diet. Low-carbohydrate diets (diets with a daily carbohydrate intake typically less than 60 g per day) have become popular since the publication of numerous diet books, the most famous of which were written by Dr Robert Atkins. There has, however, been much controversy surrounding this type of diet, with many professional organizations, including the British Dietetic Association and American Dietetic Association, cautioning against their use. The reason for this controversy is that there is a lack of research to demonstrate their safety in the long term. It has been speculated that low-carbohydrate diets may worsen blood cholesterol and triglyceride levels because lower-carbohydrate diets tend to be higher in fat. It has also been speculated that in the long term these diets may cause:

- bowel problems due to lack of fibre

- increased risk of kidney problems due to the higher protein content
- increased risk of cancer and heart disease due to the reduction in fruit and vegetable intake that some of these diets recommend.

However, no long-term studies have yet determined whether or not there is any truth in these claims.

Indeed, recent studies on low-carbohydrate diets have not only shown that the diets have no adverse effect on blood cholesterol levels, but some of the studies have even indicated that they may improve HDL-cholesterol (good cholesterol) levels and triglyceride levels. However, a more recent study found no difference in HDL-cholesterol or triglyceride levels between those who followed a low-carbohydrate diet and those who followed other reduced calorie diets for 12 months.

In 2003 a review of the research into low-carbohydrate diets was published in the *Journal of the American Medical Association*. The authors concluded that following low-carbohydrate diets will indeed help people lose weight, but that the weight loss is simply related to the reduction in overall calorie intake, not to the reduction in carbohydrate intake. In 2006, a meta-analysis of a number of studies comparing low-carbohydrate diets with low-fat diets concluded that on a low-carbohydrate diet weight loss is greater after 6 months, but that by 1 year there is no difference between low-carbohydrate and low-fat approaches.

What this means is that, if you stick to a low-carbohydrate diet, you will inevitably reduce your calorie intake and therefore lose weight. This may be due to several factors.

- If you are following a low-carbohydrate diet, you must exclude foods that are high in carbohydrates. This means that you exclude chips, cakes, crisps, chocolate, and pastries, i.e. many of the foods that are high in carbohydrates but also very high in fat (and therefore calories) and which you might have tended to overeat when not on this diet. Imagine going to a party—there are only a very small number of foods on the nibbles table which are 'allowed' on a low-carbohydrate diet, so you will automatically take in fewer calories than you would if your food choice were not so limited.
- By eating smaller amounts of carbohydrate, you will release smaller amounts of insulin and this may help you to control your cravings as well as mobilise your fat stores. Furthermore, when your diet is not providing sufficient carbohydrate to maintain your blood glucose level, you will start to use up your body's stored carbohydrate—glycogen. Once these glycogen reserves have been used up, you will burn fat as your main fuel source. Muscle

protein may be broken down and converted into glucose in order to prevent your blood glucose level from falling too low, while the breakdown of fat produces ketones which can be used by the brain when glucose is in short supply. It has been shown that these ketones may suppress the appetite, another reason why people on low-carbohydrate diets lose weight.

- When you start to eat a low-carbohydrate diet, you will soon use up your muscle and liver glycogen stores. We can store approximately 1 lb of carbohydrate in our muscles and liver. In its stored form, each gram of glycogen is attached to 3–4 g of water. When our carbohydrate intake is not adequate to maintain our blood glucose level, this carbohydrate (glycogen) is quickly used up, along with the water to which it is bound. Therefore, using up the full pound of glycogen (about 2000 calories worth) causes us to lose much more weight than we would lose by using up 2000 calories worth of fat. Because these glycogen stores account for about 4–5 lb of body weight and are used up within a couple of days, you are likely to feel initially very pleased by your rapid weight loss and this is often what encourages people to continue on this kind of diet.

See Table 19.1 for a comparison between the low-carbohydrate and low-GI dietary approaches.

What if I'm vegetarian?

A healthy low-GI diet is well suited to someone who is vegetarian. A main meal would still consist of a low-GI starchy food, plenty of vegetables, and a vegetarian source of protein. Eggs, Quorn, and soya protein are healthy choices, as they are low in fat, yet excellent sources of protein. Beans and pulses contain carbohydrate as well as protein, but are very low GI and high in fibre, so are a very nutritious low-GI food and should be eaten regularly. As for someone who is not vegetarian, dairy products must not be neglected—eat three servings per day to meet your calcium requirement. Cheese is a useful protein and calcium source, but vegetarians must take care not to rely too much on cheese as a protein source, as it is so high in saturated fat and calories.

If you are a vegan (i.e. someone who eats no animal products whatsoever), your diet may already be very restrictive. However, it is still possible to eat a balanced low-GI diet, without eating foods of animal origin. The dietary advice is the same as for vegetarians but with the exclusion of eggs and dairy products. Care should be taken to ensure that dairy substitutes are eaten three times per day and that they are fortified with calcium.

It is very difficult to adhere strictly to a low-carbohydrate diet when you do not eat meat or fish. Although Quorn and tofu contain only a small amount

Table 19.1 Low-carbohydrate versus low-GI diets

Low-GI diet	Low-carbohydrate diet
Follows healthy eating recommendations—may promote a more balanced diet	Does not follow healthy eating recommendations
High in wholegrain high-fibre foods; high in fruit and vegetables	Usually low in fibre and may be lacking in fruit and vegetables
Does not usually require supplementation	Always requires supplementation with a multivitamin and mineral preparation
Usually low in sugar and low to moderate in fat	Also low in sugar; fat usually makes up a greater proportion of calories compared with a healthy balanced diet
Can help to lower insulin levels and reduce hunger	Can help to lower insulin levels and reduce hunger
Does not lead to fat loss unless it results in a lower calorie intake	May lead to initial loss of glycogen and water stores. After this, the diet will not lead to fat loss unless it results in a lower calorie intake
No adverse effects have been reported	Side effects include constipation, dizziness, insomnia, tiredness, reduced exercise tolerance
Some high-fat foods have a low GI so may give a good impression of some unhealthy foods	Some high-fat foods are low in carbohydrate so may give a good impression of some unhealthy foods

of carbohydrate, many vegetarian and vegan protein sources, such as beans and lentils, contain a significant amount of carbohydrate, whereas meat and fish in their unprocessed form contain none. It is possible for people who are vegetarian to follow a lower-carbohydrate diet, as they have a greater variety of protein foods from which to choose. However, vegans would find their choice of foods too small if they attempted to reduce their carbohydrate intake substantially. For vegans, therefore, eating a healthy balanced diet based on low-GI carbohydrates is the practical approach.

For both vegetarians and vegans, the nutrients to take care with are as follows.

- Iron—iron from plant sources (called non-haem iron) is not absorbed as easily into the body as iron from meat sources (haem iron). Dark green vegetables and pulses are good vegetarian sources of iron. However, many other dietary components can affect how well we absorb this iron into our bodies.

- Tannins found in black tea reduce the absorption of iron.
- Calcium found in dairy products significantly decreases the absorption of iron, so dairy foods should not be eaten at the same time as good sources of non-haem iron.
- Phytates found in some unleavened breads, such as chapattis, reduce the absorption of non-haem iron.
- Vitamin C, found in fruit, vegetables, and fruit juices, helps iron to be absorbed more easily into the body, so eating a piece of fruit after a meal helps you to absorb more iron from that meal.

Iron is required for the carriage of oxygen around the body in the blood. Some women with PCOS have very heavy menstrual blood losses, and these women are at greater risk of becoming deficient in iron, which results in anaemia. Women who have heavy periods and who are vegetarian are at even greater risk. It is therefore prudent for these women to avoid drinking tea near mealtimes and instead to take fruit or fruit juice with a meal to help them absorb as much of the iron from the meal as possible.

- Protein—proteins are long molecules and are made up of 20 types of building blocks, or amino acids. Out of these 20 amino acids, eight are called 'essential' amino acids and, because the human body is unable to make them itself, we have to obtain them from our food. Animal foods contain all amino acids in the proportions that the human body requires. Plant sources of protein, however, may lack certain essential amino acids. It is therefore a good idea for people who eat few animal foods to eat a large variety of different vegetarian protein sources to ensure that they obtain all the amino acids they need. Some foods go together very well. For example, beans lack a certain amino acid of which there is an excess in bread, while bread lacks one amino acid of which there is an excess in beans. Therefore beans on toast provide a very good source of protein to meet our requirements.
- Calcium—calcium does not need to be a worry for people who eat dairy products as these are the richest source of calcium. However, vegans eat no dairy products whatsoever, so cannot take advantage of this excellent source of calcium. If you are vegan and can manage to eat three servings daily of calcium-enriched soya products, then you should be meeting your requirement for calcium. However, if you cannot manage this amount, then you should definitely consider taking a daily calcium supplement to provide 700 mg per day.

What if I eat out a lot?

Eating out poses a particular challenge for anyone who is trying to lose weight. From the moment we sit in a restaurant, we can smell the delicious aromas of the food and we can see other diners receive their delectable dishes. Bread and olives may be placed on the table, which we will start to nibble as the whole experience makes us extremely hungry. When faced with the menu, even those with very strong motivation will find it difficult to order the healthiest choice instead of the tastiest choice. Below are a few tips on how to limit the damage caused by eating out and which dishes best suit different dietary approaches to weight loss.

Tips to help you keep control

- Have a small snack just before you are leaving for the restaurant or party. Choose something light such as a piece of fruit, a bowl of sugar-free jelly, or a couple of crackers with low-fat soft cheese. This will just take the edge off your appetite, and give you a bit more control over what you order from the menu. If you feel in control when it comes to ordering, you will be more likely to pick a lower-calorie healthier dish.
- Make sure you really **taste** the food and experience how delicious it is.
- Try to eat in a similar way to the other people in the group. Always aim to be the last to finish—this will encourage you to put your fork down between mouthfuls, to savour the taste of the food rather than rushing it.
- Before the meal, decide that you will eat two courses instead of three. If you are dining with good friends or your partner, it may be helpful to share a dessert if you feel you must have one.
- Try not to drink too much alcohol with your meal, as this will reduce your ability to turn down dessert and Irish coffees!
- Remember that eating out is a very enjoyable experience. Take time to enjoy your surroundings, the conversation, the food. If you begin the occasion thinking that the meal will 'ruin your efforts' at losing weight, then it almost certainly will!

Important

It is important to remember that a low-carbohydrate diet is not nutritionally adequate and it always requires supplementation with a daily multivitamin and mineral supplement. In the first few days on a low-carbohydrate diet you will pass urine more frequently than usual, as you will be getting rid of the

Table 19.2 Lower calorie menu choices

Type of meal	Low-GI diet	Lower-carbohydrate diet
Drinks	Diet/slimline drinks or water	Diet/slimline drinks or water
Snacks	Choose sandwiches on granary bread avoiding ones drenched in mayonnaise. Eat the salad garnish	Choose a salad but leave any bread and croutons
Burger bars	Try a grilled chicken in pitta or salad now available in most chains. Alternatively try a beanburger or chickenburger	Either choose any beefburger and discard the bun, or have a chicken salad
Pub meals	Pasta or rice dish in tomato-based sauce, chilli con carne	Steak—ask for extra salad or vegetables instead of fries
Indian	Can be quite a healthy meal! Choose shashlik or tandoori dishes to avoid fatty sauces and serve with boiled basmati rice or chapatti	Choose shashlik or tandoori dishes to avoid fatty sauces. Avoid rice, naan bread, aloo dishes, and poppadums
Chinese	Chop suey, meat, or chicken in oyster sauce and stir-fried dishes are best. Serve with boiled rice or noodles	Most sauces contain a significant amount of carbohydrate and most dishes are based on rice or noodles. Stir-fried meat or prawns with vegetables is the best option
Italian	Pasta in tomato-based sauce, thick-based pizza with extra vegetables	Chicken Caesar salad or other meat or fish salad. Leave bread or croutons
Other suggestions	Choose tasty dishes, avoiding very high-fat types (pastries, dishes cooked in cream or deep-fried) and choose pasta, rice, or new potatoes to accompany	Any dish of chicken, meat, or fish without sweet sauce, breadcrumbs, or batter, served with vegetables

water that was attached to the glycogen. After this initial carbohydrate and water loss, you will start to burn off fat, which will result in the production of ketones. Although ketones are helpful in that they help suppress the appetite, they can have some less desirable side effects. In the first week of the diet, ketones may cause you to feel dizzy or light-headed on standing up. In some people, the diet may cause tiredness, whilst others have reported difficulty in sleeping. As you continue to adhere to the diet, these symptoms will improve or disappear. Ketones do have a distinctive smell (like pear drops or nail varnish remover) which may be detected faintly on the breath. In order to minimize the effects of ketones and to ensure that you keep your kidneys working properly, it is vital that you drink at least 2 litres of fluids per day if you choose to follow a lower-carbohydrate diet.

Meal replacements

The term 'meal replacements' is used to describe products used to replace meals to aid weight control. They are usually in the form of a vitamin- and mineral-enriched milkshake drink or meal bar, and are designed to provide a balanced nutrient intake in a controlled number of calories. The best known of these are produced by Slim·Fast. The idea is that the 'dieter' has two meal replacement products per day, replacing breakfast and lunch. They are encouraged to have a snack of fruit or a meal replacement snack bar mid-morning and mid-afternoon and then to have a well-balanced 600 calorie meal in the evening.

There has been some reasonable research demonstrating that this approach to weight loss works in both the short and longer term. In one such paper, the investigators studied 100 overweight and moderately obese men and women, whom they randomized into two groups. For the first 3 months, group A were given advice to follow a traditional 1200–1500 calorie diet whilst group B were given two meal replacements per day and advised to eat a 700–800 calorie meal. For the following 4 years, both groups were put on the same regime—to have one meal replacement per day and to eat two sensible meals of 500 and 700 calories. Both groups of patients were followed for 51 months, monitored monthly, and given the meal replacement products free of charge.

Figure 19.1 shows that people taking the meal replacement products twice a day (group B) lost considerably more weight in the first 3 months than those who were not using any meal replacement products. Furthermore, the rate at which group B lost weight actually increased from 3 months onwards, following the introduction of one meal replacement per day. However, the subjects involved in this research may have been more inclined to comply with the regime than people who have to pay for the meal replacement products. It is also worth bearing in mind that this research was funded by Slim·Fast!

One of the reasons that meal replacement products might help people lose weight is that they enable people to consume fewer calories without having to spend time planning all their meals—most of the calories are counted for you. When making a meal, one person's idea of a 'portion' might be quite different from another person's 'portion'. With meal replacements, the portion

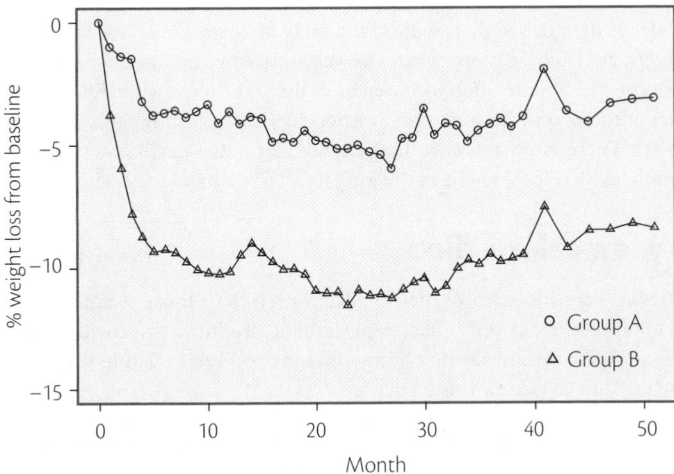

Figure 19.1 Comparison of percentage of body weight loss by those using meal replacements compared with those consuming a 1200–1500 calorie diet. From Flechtner-Mors M *et al.* (2000) Metabolic and weight loss effects of long-term dietary intervention in obese patients: four-year results. *Obesity Research* 8: 399–402.

size is predetermined and there aren't any leftovers for second helpings. Meal replacements may be particularly useful for people who are always on the go or who don't have much time to prepare meals. If we are faced with too much choice, we often find it difficult to select the lowest calorie or healthiest foods. Using meal replacements eliminates this choice and therefore may help people to avoid the situations that lead to overeating. Most experts in weight management are of the opinion that people are more likely to lose weight if they follow a structured type of eating plan. However, the guidance on the management of obesity recently published by the government's National Institute for Clinical Excellence found inadequate evidence that there was any benefit in using meal replacements over and above other forms of calorie-controlled diet.

Typically, women following a meal replacement plan consume around 1400 calories per day. This would allow the majority of women to lose at least 1 lb of fat per week. Furthermore, the milkshake drinks have a low GI, and so should help keep insulin levels down, and may help to reduce feelings of hunger later in the day. As with any weight loss plan, it is important that lifestyle changes are maintained in the long term to prevent the weight being regained.

Detox diets

The idea is that 'detox' diets will rid the body of 'toxins' (alcohol, caffeine, food additives, etc.). These diets tend to be very restrictive and are not intended for long-term use. People often lose weight in the short term when following these diets, but this is only because they restrict calories by cutting out so many types of foods. There is no evidence that eliminating foods in this way will make a person healthier, lose weight in the long term, or detoxify the body.

Very low calorie diets

The term 'very low calorie diet' or VLCD refers to those weight loss plans on which people eat only meal replacement products to provide a total of less than 800 calories per day. These include products such as Lighter Life, Lipotrim, and the Cambridge Diet.

These diets are designed to promote weight loss of around 3 lb per week. However, they are extremely restrictive and require the 'dieter' to eat only the meal replacement products provided—no other food is allowed. Usually your doctor is required to request the 'prescription' of these diets, and regular medical checks are recommended throughout the diet. The reason for this is that such rapid weight loss can have some undesirable effects on the body.

- Although weight is lost quickly, a large proportion of this is due to loss of muscle tissue, including heart muscle.
- Losing weight too quickly can cause an increase in uric acid levels in the blood which causes gout.

Although there is no doubt that these diets produce weight loss, there is little evidence to suggest that people keep the weight off when normal food is reintroduced. These diets need to be followed alongside behavioural therapy and counselling to help the dieter learn how to change their eating habits in the long term.

VLCDs might seem like an ideal quick-fix solution to someone's weight problem, but they could merely reinforce the 'all-or-nothing' thinking that caused the dieter to become overweight in the first place. Likewise, they might reinforce the unrealistic goals that yo-yo dieters have of losing weight—people lose lean tissue very quickly on VLCD programmes, so might expect to lose fat at the same rate and be disappointed when this doesn't happen. Also there is little more depressing than restricting yourself to peculiar-tasting drinks for weeks on end, losing a few stone and then putting it all back on within a couple of months!

It is important to remember that different approaches to losing weight suit different people. There is no one approach that will work for everyone. The bottom line is that you will only lose fat if you are taking in fewer calories than you burn off. If you restrict your intake too much, you are likely to overeat more when you inevitably do give in to temptation. If you would like to talk to an expert about your diet or have any questions about alternative dietary approaches, then ask your doctor or nurse to refer you to a registered dietitian. Dietitians are uniquely qualified to translate scientific information about food into practical dietary advice. The title dietitian can only be used by those appropriately trained professionals who have registered with the Health Professions Council, so you can be assured that you will receive reliable advice and information.

20

Behavioural aspects of losing weight

 Key points

- People who are trying to lose weight often think in an 'all or nothing' way about food. This leads to a cycle of restriction followed by overeating, which causes weight gain and further reduces self esteem.
- Food is used as a comfort when we are bored, stressed, or upset. It may be useful in these situations to consider whether the food really does make you feel better.
- There are several strategies which we can use to help us gain control of our eating or to help us develop a more positive relationship with food.

If everybody ate only when they were hungry, then very few of us would be overweight. There are many situations and emotions that cause us to eat whether we are hungry or not.

- We may use food and drink to treat or reward ourselves.
- We often eat because we are bored.
- We often eat when we are stressed.
- We may use food as a comfort when we feel unhappy or depressed.
- If we feel bad about ourselves we might use food as a punishment.
- We often choose particular foods and drinks to signify a celebration.
- If someone else has given us food as a treat or gift, we feel we should share the treat there and then rather than put it away for another time.
- Social gatherings often revolve entirely around food and drink.

- We sometimes associate a particular activity with eating, for example we would probably eat popcorn at the cinema even if it is 10 p.m.

The rest of this chapter describes some techniques that you can try to help you overcome some problem eating behaviours. Whichever way you choose to reduce your calorie intake and increase your energy expenditure, we would strongly suggest that you use some of these strategies as part of your long-term weight loss plan.

Cognitive change: changing your attitude to food

Many overweight people have tried numerous 'diets'. Each diet has a different set of strict rules. What we suggest is that you now teach yourself to think differently. Working within flexible guidelines instead of strict rules will allow you to cope better in a situation where the rules are broken.

Eating is associated with a huge range of emotions and situations. At the same time our society is very preoccupied with weight, and our culture causes us to dislike our bodies by portraying unrealistic images of body shapes and sizes in magazines, television, and celebrities.

Therefore, more often than not, when we eat for any reason other than because it is a mealtime, the enjoyment of eating is shortly followed by guilt, particularly if the food we ate was high in calories. The feelings of guilt might cause us to think that we have lost control and that we have failed. People who are trying to lose weight often think in a very 'all-or-nothing' kind of way about foods and dieting. While they are 'on a diet' they restrict their food intake considerably, and are often heard saying things like

> I'm never eating chocolate again

or

> I'm always going to have fruit for pudding.

Dichotomous thinking

Imagine you are at home and you are 'on a diet' and as part of your 'diet' you have decided you are not going to eat any chocolate …

- After a week of eating like a sparrow, you arrive home late, tired, and stressed out by the day you've had and you are craving chocolate.
- You take a chocolate bar out of the cupboard and eat it to comfort yourself but you eat it quickly because you aren't supposed to have it.

- As soon as you've eaten it you begin to feel guilty because you weren't supposed to be eating any chocolate.
- You think 'I've ruined it now' and you feel that you've lost control.
- Then you think that you might as well have another chocolate bar seeing as you've ruined your 'diet' anyway.
- Having eaten two chocolate bars, you feel terribly guilty and feel like you've totally lost control. So you then decide to finish **all** the chocolate bars in the house so that you can start all over again with **none** left in the house from tomorrow.

As you can see from this example, it is possible to have very negative feelings towards foods such as chocolate simply because they are perceived as being 'bad' foods and ones which are not allowed when we are 'on a diet'. This causes us to have very dichotomous (all-or-nothing, black-or-white, good-or-bad) thinking about the food. The end result of this thought process is that, instead of having one chocolate bar and enjoying it, you end up eating five chocolate bars and feeling terrible about it.

Do you think you might ever be in the situation where you eat some delicious pineapple and then think that you'd better eat another five pineapples so that you can start again with none tomorrow? It's very unlikely because, as tasty as pineapples may be, you won't feel guilty for eating it, so it won't cause you to think in such an all-or-nothing way about it. We're not suggesting that you swap all chocolate for pineapples (!); we're simply suggesting that you learn to enjoy chocolate, just like thin women do, and not feel guilty for eating it.

Many of the women I see in the PCOS clinic have a very distorted view of certain foods. They tend to place high-calorie foods high up on a pedestal, as they believe that these are foods which they should not be eating. They may believe that they do not deserve to eat these foods. They believe that only lucky slim women are able to eat chocolate, cakes, and biscuits, and that they themselves are not worthy of these high-calorie foods as they need to lose weight.

These women are the same women who will eat the last chocolate in the tin, even if it's the strawberry cream one that everyone else has avoided, just because it's chocolate, so it must be nice, mustn't it? They are also the same women who will panic when someone at work brings in a cake—even before they find out what sort of cake it is. They assume that because something is high in calories, it must be delicious and therefore they will not be able to help themselves when offered it ... and once they've had one piece they might lose all control and have some more ...

What we would like you to do is this: when faced with the offer of a food which is high in calories, visualize it being lowered down from its pedestal. Instead of thinking that you are not worthy of eating this food, think instead whether the food in question is actually good enough for you. If there is one chocolate left over in the tin from Christmas, instead of eating it straight away, consider why it is the only one left. Is it really that nice? Is it one of your favourite chocolates? Compare how you think it will taste with how good your favourite food tastes. Is it going to be anywhere near as nice as your favourite food? Were you just going to eat it because no one else wants it? If so, do you normally treat yourself like a dustbin?

Remember that, as we explained in Chapter 13, the greater your self-esteem, the more likely you are to have the motivation you need to lose weight. Treating yourself like a dustbin will not help you to build your self-esteem.

Comfort eating

It is not unusual for people to use food as a comfort, particularly when they are bored or unhappy. Many people have been brought up considering certain foods to be treats or rewards. Parents can often be heard telling their children that if they are good then they can have some chocolate or go to McDonalds. It is unsurprising, therefore, that we might treat ourselves with unhealthy foods given the chance.

If you are concerned that your comfort eating is stopping you losing weight, then you could try some of these techniques.

1. When you are bored or unhappy at home and you are about to go to the kitchen to have a look for some food, consider the following.
   - When you normally go to look for food, what normally happens?
   - Think about what it was that you wanted the food to do. Were you going to eat because you were bored or upset, etc.?
   - Now consider whether this food will do the job that you want it to do. How will you feel after you have eaten it? If you are bored, once you've eaten the food will your boredom have miraculously disappeared? If you are upset, do you think you will feel better about yourself after eating that food?
   - Only do things that make you feel good about yourself. If eating that food will make you feel better about yourself, then eat it. If food is not going to do the job, think of something that will—whether it's applying fake tan and painting your nails, or finally getting through that pile of ironing that's been making you feel bad every time you look at it.
2. Have you ever eaten a large portion of popcorn at the cinema whilst watching a film? Would you eat that much popcorn at home if you were sitting at

the dinner table? Research has shown that watching television causes people to consume significantly more calories than they would do if they were not watching television. The most likely reason for this is that people eat more when they are not concentrating on what they are eating. Try the following techniques to help you eat less without even noticing that you are eating less.

- Whenever you are eating anything—whether it be a meal, a snack, or something as small as an after-dinner mint—taste it as though you are a food critic. Imagine you have to write a review about the food after you've eaten it, so that you really concentrate on the taste, smell, and feel of the food. This is easier to do if you slow down your eating to allow you to savour each mouthful. Make sure that you aren't reloading your fork until you have finished your previous mouthful—whilst there is food in your mouth you should be concentrating on that food, not on scooping up the next mouthful.
- You can't concentrate properly on the taste of your food if you are driving, working on the computer, watching television, or reading at the same time. If you have to eat your dinner in front of the television, just make sure that all of your concentration is focused on the food, not the television.
- By focusing more on the food, you will develop a more positive relationship with food. You may discover that some foods aren't actually as tasty as you thought they were, so you can move towards eating only the foods that are truly delicious and which are worthy of you eating them.

It is important to remember to eat foods that you find delicious. Women who are trying to lose weight sometimes convince themselves that they like certain foods just because they are perceived to be healthy. A few women with PCOS have proudly told me that every time they have had a craving for chocolate, they have eaten a bowl of muesli instead. When I asked them what happened when they did this, they told me that they often felt unsatisfied so ate a second bowl of muesli. When I asked what happened after this, they all said that they eventually gave in and ate the chocolate. So instead of just eating 250 calories worth of chocolate and enjoying it, they had eaten 600 calories worth of muesli followed by 250 calories worth of chocolate, which they then felt guilty about. Although muesli is much healthier than chocolate, 850 calories are a lot more fattening than 250!

Eating when you are already full

Many people have been brought up to finish everything that is on their plate. They were not allowed pudding unless they had finished their main course, and they were not allowed to leave the table until their plate was clean.

Unfortunately, this has caused many people to lose the sensation of being full. Some people do notice when their stomachs feel full but still continue eating anyway until their eyes inform them that their plate is empty. However large the portion, we somehow manage to fit it in. This is particularly true if a new food is offered, such as a dessert. Consider the following points if you are someone who finds it difficult to leave food on their plate.

1. What was the reason that you were asked to finish everything that was on your plate? Was it because your parents grew up at a time when food was rationed so they were taught to eat everything they were given? Was it because there were starving children in Ethiopia who would give anything for that food? Or was it because you were the youngest child and your older siblings would have eaten it all if you didn't eat it first?

   If you feel that it is wasteful to leave food imagine this.

   You are starving child in Ethiopia. You are lucky if you have a little porridge or leaves to eat a couple of times a week. Imagine that you see a slim woman in Britain discarding a bit of food at the end of her meal.

   Now imagine you are watching a very overweight woman in Britain patting her stomach after a large roast dinner and puffing and panting as she says 'Goodness I am so stuffed but I'm just going to finish this last potato'.

   Is either of them less wasteful than the other? Does either of them make the starving child in Ethiopia feel any less hungry?

   It is important to challenge our beliefs about food. Britain is not short of food. There is an abundance of food, especially convenient high-calorie food. So it might be time to reconsider what we mean by 'wasteful'.

2. If you taste everything you eat as though you are a food critic, you will feel much more satisfied by what you are eating. When you get to the point in the meal at which it is more of a struggle to eat than a pleasure, then that's the time to save the rest for later. If you don't, you are likely to finish the meal and feel uncomfortably full. You might then feel guilty for eating so much and so you may even have a high-calorie snack later because you are having a 'bad day' so might as well eat loads and start the diet again tomorrow!

3. Do you save the best bit until last? Despite being a sign of intelligence, saving the best bit of a meal until the end won't help you to lose weight. However full you are, you will still force down the last mouthfuls because they are, by your own definition, the best bits. If you want to learn to stop when you're full, then start eating the best bits first.

Problem-solving

Problem-solving is where you try to pre-empt a problem situation or behaviour and figure out ways to help you deal with it. You can apply this technique to any problem to help you find the most realistic way of solving it, in the same way that Karen does below.

Karen's problem

Karen thinks her problem is that she eats too many biscuits when she's bored at home. She does the food shopping each week and buys several packets of chocolate biscuits because her partner wants them.

Step 1: Identifying the problem

I need to have biscuits in the house for my partner and I think I may be eating too many of them myself.

Step 2: Stating the problem accurately

I have looked at my food diary and I've noticed that on most days I'm eating 3–7 biscuits, which I only buy because my partner wants them.

Step 3: Thinking of as many solutions as possible

- I could just stop buying them altogether and see if he notices.
- I could carry on buying them and try harder not to eat them.
- I could ask him if he could take his biscuits to work so I don't see them.
- I could buy him biscuits that I don't like.

Step 4: Deciding which solution is most realistic and practical

- I can't stop buying them because he has told me that he'd feel deprived.
- I know that I don't have the willpower to not eat them if I see them.
- I think the most realistic approach is to ask my partner to buy his own favourite biscuits for him to have only at work. I'll buy one pack of biscuits that I don't really like for him to have at home—that way I won't be tempted to eat biscuits in the house.

Step 5: Trying out the solution and establishing whether or not it helped

If the chosen solution is not successful, try a different approach next time it happens.

The important thing to remember about this problem-solving technique is that only you will know which solution will work best for you. Remember, what works for one person does not necessarily work for another.

Stimulus control

If it's not there I can't eat it

Stimulus control means finding ways to avoid a situation that makes you tempted to overeat. That means removing the tempting food from the area around you, so that you don't think about it so often. It may also mean avoiding other cues to eat. For example, if you eat a pie every time you go to a football match or you eat a large carton of popcorn every time you go to the cinema, it may be helpful to limit these outings whilst you are trying to lose weight.

Shopping to a list and shopping on a full stomach are also important tips to remember to help control the temptation to make less healthy food choices. If the smell of food in a shop or supermarket tempts you to overeat, then try to avoid going near that shop. Doing your weekly supermarket shop on the Internet is a very useful means of avoiding the many stimuli that are present in supermarkets. By doing your shopping online you can ensure that you shop at a time when you are not hungry. You avoid being faced with shelves full of high-calorie treats on 'special offer', and you also avoid having the wonderfully tempting smell of freshly baked bread making you suddenly feel ravenous.

Urge surfing

I'll eat it if I still want it in 5 minutes time

This can be particularly helpful to people who eat impulsively in response to emotions or mood, and it is very simple. The idea is that when you feel the urge to eat outside of a planned meal, delay eating for a while, initially for 5 minutes. So when you are watching TV in the evening and you feel the urge to grab a couple of biscuits, think to yourself:

> I'll just wait for 5 minutes. If, after 5 minutes, I still want the biscuits then I can have them, but I'll see how I feel in 5 minutes' time.

During the 5 minute wait, you could do something to pass the time, such as make a cup of tea or brush your teeth. When the 5 minutes is up, reassess how you feel. The chances are that you will feel empowered by the fact that you could wait for that 5 minutes and you'll decide not to eat the biscuits. However, if you do still want the biscuits, it is no problem, just make sure you serve up two biscuits on a plate and put the rest of the packet back in the cupboard. Eat them slowly and savour the taste of them, as you must take the time to enjoy them. Biscuits are tasty and are made to be enjoyed, so you should not feel guilty for eating a couple occasionally. All too often we forget to concentrate on the food that is in our mouth, as we are too preoccupied with feeling guilty about eating it. Remember to taste what is in your mouth at the time and enjoy it.

Behaviour chains

Behaviour chain diagrams can be very useful for helping people get to the root of their eating problem. If there are times when you are particularly likely to overeat, then it may be worth drawing yourself a diagram of exactly what is going on, just like the one shown in Fig. 20.1. In any behaviour chain there are three parts.

1. Antecedents—the events that trigger the behaviour
2. Behaviours
3. Consequences—what happens as a result of the behaviour

In the example in Fig. 20.1, the antecedents include:

- Getting up late
- Skipping breakfast
- Being at home mid-morning tired and bored
- Seeing the biscuits when making a cup of tea

The behaviours include:

- Eating two biscuits whilst making a cup of tea (not concentrating on biscuits)
- Bringing the packet through into the lounge
- Eating four more biscuits whilst watching TV (not concentrating on biscuits)
- Feeling guilty about it and feeling like she's ruined her diet so she might as well finish the packet (all-or-nothing thinking).

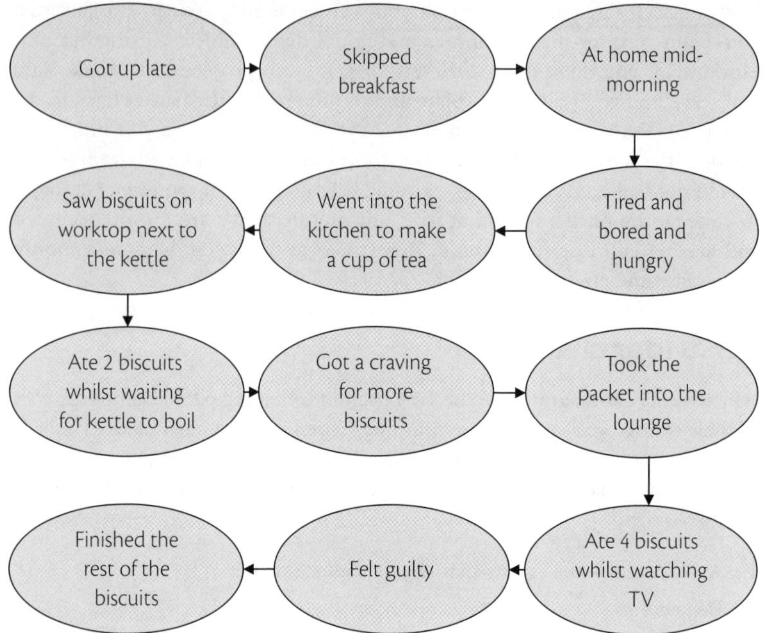

Figure 20.1 Example of a behaviour chain.

The consequence is that she's eaten a whole packet of biscuits.

By putting this diagram down on paper, it becomes clear which stages of this process could be done differently next time to avoid this happening again. As with all aspects of weight management, different things suit different people. Whereas one woman might choose to start having breakfast to avoid being hungry mid-morning, another might find this very difficult and prefer to store the biscuits in a high cupboard and go for a walk to get out of the house mid-morning. Someone else might choose to use the urge-surfing technique when they get a craving for biscuits whilst making a cup of tea.

Hopefully this chapter has helped you identify some of your troublesome eating behaviours and has given you some ideas as to how you might begin to change your behaviour and attitude towards food.

21

Your individual weight loss plan

Key points

- It is best not to begin trying to lose weight until you have made the necessary preparations described in this chapter.
- Calculating how many calories you expend will give you a firm basis on which to build your individualised weight loss plan.
- Use whichever dietary approaches suit you to help you eat your recommended calorie intake, as long as the diet is nutritionally adequate.

To create your own individual weight loss plan, follow the steps below. It is important to complete all the steps in order, as this will increase your chance of success.

Step 1: Make sure the time is right

This step may last any length of time from 30 minutes to 30 years! It is vital that you wait until your weight is a priority for you and you are absolutely ready to dedicate time and effort into losing weight. If you are unsure whether the time is right, make a list of the pros and cons of losing weight and of not losing weight (see Table 13.1 on page 103).

Step 2: Be prepared

1. Prepare and keep an accurate food and activity diary.

   Whilst making an effort to eat your typical diet, start keeping a food and activity diary. Use the example diary in Appendix 1 for ideas and see Chapter 17 for information on how to make the most out of keeping your diary.

Table 21.1 Equations to estimate an individual's energy expenditure

Age	BMR for women	BMR for men
10–18 years	12.2 × weight in kg + 746	17.5 × weight in kg + 651
18–30 years	14.7 × weight in kg + 496	15.3 × weight in kg + 679
30–60 years	8.7 × weight in kg + 829	11.6 × weight in kg + 879
>60 years	10.5 × weight in kg + 596	13.5 × weight in kg + 487

2. Analyse your own food diary.

   Look back over your food diary and see if there are any obvious problems with your eating behaviour. For example, are you skipping meals early in the day resulting in overeating later in the evening? You might want to set yourself some SMART goals to help normalize your eating behaviour. See Chapter 17 for more information about goal setting.

3. Prepare a progress chart

   Prepare yourself a chart or book for keeping a weekly record of your weight and various measurements. There is an example progress chart in Appendix 2.

4. Calculate your energy expenditure

   Energy expenditure is calculated by finding out your basal metabolic rate (BMR) and multiplying it by your physical activity level (PAL). Your BMR can be quite accurately estimated using the calculations in Table 21.1. Although this book is for women with PCOS, we have included the calculations for men in case you are trying to lose weight with your partner.

Once you have calculated your BMR, you need to multiply it by your PAL (Table 21.2). For most people, the PAL will be 1.3, as this assumes a normal sedentary day without any particular exercise. Someone who works in an office and does not do any structured exercise would fit this category.

- Light activity assumes some daily exercise at work or tasks about the house or garden with at least 2 hours on your feet. Someone who works as a cleaner for a few hours per day would fit this category.
- Moderate activity assumes 6 hours on your feet per day or regular strenuous exercise. For example, a busy nurse or waitress would fit this category.
- Heavy activity is for people in heavy labouring jobs or serious athletes in training. A painter/decorator or distance runner would fit this category.

Table 21.2 Physical activity levels (PALs) for women and men

Activity level	PAL for women	PAL for men
Inactive	1.3	1.3
Light	1.56	1.55
Moderate	1.64	1.78
Heavy	1.82	2.1

Alternatively you can calculate your estimated energy requirement based on an 'inactive' PAL and add on the calories you use up through activity by using the table in Appendix 3.

For example, a 28-year-old woman, weighing 89 kg, drives to her office to work and goes to a 50 minute aerobics class twice a week, but 10 minutes of the class is taken up by stretching.

Weight = 89 kg PAL = 1.3

BMR = 15.3 × 89 + 679 = 2040 calories

Daily energy expenditure = 2040 × 1.3 = 2652 calories

She therefore burns off 2652 calories per day without exercising. She works out that she burns off an extra 400 calories per aerobics session, i.e. 800 calories per week. When this is spread out over 7 days, it means she burns off an additional 115 calories each day, so her total energy expenditure is 2767 calories per day.

Use Appendix 3 to add on an appropriate number of calories for any regular physical activity you do.

5. Work out how much you should be eating

   We know that we need to burn off 3500 calories more than we are eating in order to lose 1 lb of body fat, so Table 21.3 explains what you should be eating in order to lose weight. It shows the quantity of each of the different food groups that you should be aiming to eat in order to have a healthy balanced diet within a specified number of calories.

To use the table, you simply look up your energy expenditure in the column on the left-hand side. Once you have found your own energy expenditure in the table, you can establish how much you should be eating by using the information in the other columns relating to your own energy expenditure. The

Table 21.3 Guidelines for dietary intake to lose weight

Your energy expenditure	Calorie prescription for weight loss	To lose 1 lb of fat every …	Fruit and vegetables	Bread, cereals, and starchy foods	Meat, fish, and alternatives	Milk and dairy products	Fats	Actual energy value of these portions	Allowance for extras
1700	1500	17 days	5	7	2	2	2	1360	140
1800	1500	11 days	5	7	2	2	2	1360	140
1900	1500	9 days	5	7	2	2	2	1360	140
2000	1500	1 week	5	7	2	2	2	1360	140
2100	1600	1 week	6	7	2	3	2	1490	110
2200	1700	1 week	7	8	2	3	2	1610	90
2300	1800	1 week	7	8	3	3	2	1760	40
2400	1900	1 week	7	8	3	3	3	1820	80
2500	2000	1 week	8	8	3	3	3	1860	140
2600	2100	1 week	8	9	3	3	4	2000	100

2700	2200	1 week	8	9	4	3	4	2150	50
2800	1800	1/2 week	7	8	3	3	2	1760	40
2900	1900	1/2 week	7	8	3	3	3	1820	80
3000	2000	1/2 week	8	8	3	3	3	1860	140
3100	2100	1/2 week	8	9	3	3	4	2000	100
3200	2200	1/2 week	8	9	4	3	4	2150	50
3300	2300	1/2 week	9	9	4	3	4	2190	110
3400	2400	1/2 week	9	9	4	4	4	2280	120
3500	2500	1/2 week	10	9	4	4	5	2380	120
3600	2600	1/2 week	10	10	4	4	5	2460	140
3700	2700	1/2 week	11	10	4	4	5	2500	200

second and third columns explain how many calories you need to be eating in order to lose weight and how quickly the weight will be lost if you eat this recommended number of calories. The other columns show how many units you should eat from each food group in order to eat the recommended number of calories.

Going back to the previous example, a woman who burns off 2767 calories each day would look up 2800 calories on the left-hand column of the table. By looking across that row on the table she can see that she will lose 2 lb of fat each week by eating 1800 calories per day. (If she preferred to eat 500 more calories and lose weight at half the rate, she could choose to follow the portions guide for a 2300 calorie diet and therefore lose 1 lb per week.)

5. Prepare yourself a portions checklist

   Keeping a checklist helps you keep track of how many portions you have used and therefore how much of your allowance you have left for the rest of the day. For example, if you were aiming to eat 1500 calories per day, you would look up your 1500 calorie diet in Table 21.3 and then make a checklist of the prescribed portions like that shown in Table 21.4. If you prepare your checklist on a computer, you can print off seven copies of your daily checklist each week.

Step 3: Do it

Now you are ready to go ahead and follow the plan that you have designed to fit your needs.

Table 21.4 Daily portions checklist for a 1500 calorie diet plan

Fruit and vegetables	Bread, other cereals, and potatoes	Meat, fish, and alternatives	Milk and dairy products	Fats	Extras allowance
F	B	Mt	Mk	Fat	140 calories
F	B	Mt	Mk	Fat	
F	B				
F	B				
F	B				
F	B				
F	B				

1. Start filling in your progress chart. Measure your weight not more often than once a week and try to do this at the same time each week, at a time when you believe your weight should be similar each time (i.e. try 8 a.m. on a Thursday rather than 2 p.m. on a Sunday!).

2. Monitor your food intake and energy expenditure by continuing to keep your food, mood, and activity diary.

3. Start to work towards developing healthy eating behaviour by analysing your own food diary and using the information in Chapter 20 of this book. If you do not currently eat breakfast, taking the first steps towards making breakfast a habit might be the most helpful change you could possibly make towards managing your weight in the long term.

4. You should by now have incorporated some physical activity into your lifestyle to increase your energy expenditure, your confidence, and your self-esteem.

5. When you eat a food, use the tables in Appendix 4 to see how many 'units' that food is worth. For example, if the first thing you eat in the morning is six tablespoons of Special K with milk, you would see in Appendix 4 that three tablespoons of Special K is one unit of 'bread, cereals, and potatoes', so, by having six tablespoons, you are eating two units. The milk is equivalent to one unit of 'milk and dairy foods', so you would mark your whole breakfast off on your checklist as in Table 21.5.

Table 21.5 Using the checklist to mark off one bowl of cereal with milk

Fruit and vegetables	Bread, other cereals and potatoes	Meat, fish and alternatives	Milk and dairy products	Fats	Extras allowance
F	~~B~~	Mt	~~Mk~~	Fat	140 calories
F	~~B~~	Mt	Mk	Fat	
F	B				
F	B				
F	B				
F	B				
F	B				

For lunch you might have a tuna sandwich with a small bowl of salad on the side, a glass of orange juice, and a nectarine to follow. You would need to look up the following items in Appendix 4:

- 2 slices of medium-thick bread
- 2 tsp of low-fat spread
- 1 tin of tuna in brine
- 1 small bowl of salad
- 1 nectarine
- 1 small glass of orange juice

Your updated checklist would then look like Table 21.6.

Table 21.6 Using your checklist to mark off lunch

Fruit and vegetables	Bread, other cereals, and potatoes	Meat, fish, and alternatives	Milk and dairy products	Fats	Extras allowance
~~F~~	~~B~~	~~Mt~~	~~Mk~~	~~Fat~~	140 calories
~~F~~	~~B~~	Mt	Mk	Fat	
~~F~~	~~B~~				
F	~~B~~				
F	B				
F	B				
F	B				

You can then decide how you are going to eat during the rest of the day. If, for example, you were planning to have chilli and rice for your evening meal, you can choose whether or not to use up all of your remaining three 'bread, other cereals, and potatoes' portions on the rice alone. The table in Appendix 4 tells you that two tablespoons of boiled rice are equivalent to one unit. Therefore, you could use up all three remaining 'bread, cereals, and potatoes' portions by having six tablespoons of boiled rice with your chilli. Or you might choose to have four tablespoons of rice, so that you can plan to have a slice of toast later in the evening if that's when you tend to get a little peckish.

6. In order to keep your cravings at bay and to keep your insulin levels as low as possible, incorporate low-GI diet principles into your eating plan. This will make it easier for you to reduce your calorie intake than it would do if you ate a high-GI diet, which would trigger those dreaded carbohydrate cravings. Familiarize yourself with Chapter 18 of this book and use the GI table in Appendix 6 as a reference to help you adopt a lower-GI diet. You can use the GI table to help you decide which foods to choose from the 'bread, other cereals, and potatoes' section. Don't forget that including plenty of protein with your meal will reduce the GI of the whole meal, even if the meal includes your favourite high-GI food such as mashed potato or French bread!

   If there are certain foods which you know pose a particular problem for you, then feel free to adapt the diet so that it suits you. Some women with PCOS find it easier to lose weight eating a diet that's lower in carbohydrate, so they might choose to adapt the portions on their plan to reflect this, for example by reducing their 'bread, cereals, and potatoes' portions by three (80 calories each) and adding one 'meat, fish, and alternatives' portion (150 calories) and one 'dairy' portion (90 calories). In this way, the resulting plan provides the same number of calories but suits that particular woman better. Please note, however, that the prescribed portions given in Table 21.3 are based on the proportions of a balanced diet (Fig. 14.1). Any deviation from these suggested plans will result in your diet being less well balanced based on recommendations set by the leading nutritional authorities in the UK.

7. Be flexible. All of these steps require effort to complete, even if that effort is just remembering to weigh yourself or fill in a food diary. Remember to take things one step at a time and not try to change everything at once. Revisit your first food diary and look at your eating behaviour. It may be important for you to learn to eat high-calorie foods without feeling guilty, so don't worry if at first your diet is not perfectly balanced. Once you have developed a more positive relationship with food, the time will come for you to work on the overall balance of your diet and lifestyle.

8. Remember your realistic expectations.

   - You can only lose a pound of fat if you have eaten 3500 calories less than you have burnt off.

- People usually lose weight for 12–15 weeks so build this fact into your plan. After 12–15 weeks, you need to change tactics and actively try to keep your weight the same, at least for a month, before you attempt to lose any more weight. For information about this, see Chapter 22 of this book.

Summary

1. Once you have established that this is the right time for you to be focusing on losing weight, you can start to make preparations.
2. Prepare yourself a food, mood, and activity diary and begin to fill it in before you start to change your eating habits.
3. Analyse your food diary to see if there are any problems with your eating behaviour that are likely to hinder your efforts to lose weight.
4. Prepare yourself a progress chart to keep a record of your achievements as you begin to make changes to your lifestyle.
5. Calculate how many calories you burn off each day, including those used up in regular physical activity, using Tables 21.1 and 21.2 as well as Appendix 3.
6. Work out how much food you should be eating to lose weight, using the portions guide in Table 21.3.
7. Make yourself a checklist of your diet plan, like that shown in Table 21.4, to help you keep to the correct number of portions. Cross off the portions as you eat them.
8. Make the effort to swap some high-GI foods with lower-GI types. This will make it easier for you to keep to your calorie-controlled diet.
9. Think flexibly about your plan and always remember what you can realistically be expected to achieve.

22

Treatment of obesity: the role of drugs and surgery

Key points

- There are currently three drugs which are licensed for use in the UK for the treatment of obesity. All require a doctor's prescription and are only licensed for adults with a BMI>30kg/m^2.
- Approximately 50–60% of individuals who change their diet, increase their physical activity, and take obesity medication will lose 5–10 per cent of their body weight.
- In women who are extremely overweight who have tried lifestyle measures and prescription medication with little success, weight loss surgery may be the final option. Although many obesity-related problems resolve after surgery, it is not to be undertaken lightly as there is a significant risk of complications.

Obesity is defined as the accumulation of excess fat resulting in a body weight which is more than 25 per cent above what is considered to be normal for sex and height. The body mass index (BMI) is the measure most often used to determine whether someone is obese. You are obese if your BMI is greater than 30. The number of people in the Western world who are obese has soared over the past 30 years, and currently about a third of all adults in the USA and just under a quarter of adults in the UK are obese. Being obese increases your risks of developing diseases such as diabetes and heart disease. However, the good news is that by losing only 5–10 per cent of your initial weight, for example 20 lb if you weigh 200 lb, you can significantly reduce the risk of disease associated with being obese. Many people find it difficult to lose weight and keep the weight off. Consequently there has been a lot of research into the use of medication and surgery in the treatment of obesity.

Anti-obesity drugs

There are currently three drugs which are licensed for use in the UK for the treatment of obesity. The drugs will only work when combined with a change in diet and an increase in physical activity. At best the drugs will enhance your weight loss efforts if you have already changed your lifestyle to include a healthy diet and regular physical activity. The drugs are only available on a doctor's prescription and can only be prescribed if your BMI is over 30, or over 28 if you have diabetes or another obesity-related complication.

Orlistat (Xenical)

Orlistat prevents the absorption of fat from your diet by inhibiting the enzyme needed to digest it. This in turn reduces the number of calories absorbed by the body, resulting in weight loss. Trials have shown that people taking orlistat lose on average 4 kg (9 lb) more than those not on orlistat and over half will lose 5–10 per cent of their body weight. Orlistat has also been shown to reduce the risk of developing diabetes in high-risk individuals and to reduce cholesterol levels. You need to stick to a low-fat diet while taking orlistat otherwise the unabsorbed fat causes diarrhoea, oily stool, bloating, flatulence, and sometimes faecal urgency or incontinence. These side effects are uncommon if you are on a low-fat diet.

Sibutramine (Reductil or Merida)

This drug acts by blocking the action of two chemicals in the brain, noradrenaline and serotonin. These chemicals are involved in appetite regulation, so blocking their action makes you feel full more quickly so that you eat less and lose weight. Sibutramine may also increase your metabolic rate, resulting in an increase in calories burned. Clinical trials have shown that approximately 75 per cent of patients taking sibutramine will lose 5 per cent of their initial body weight. People on sibutramine lose on average 4 kg (9 lb) more than those not taking the drug. Side effects include headaches, dry mouth, constipation, insomnia, and an increase in heart rate and blood pressure. You should not take sibutramine if you are pregnant or are seeking pregnancy, if you have uncontrolled high blood pressure, heart disease, or a mental illness, or you are taking antidepressants. Finally, when you first start taking sibutramine you will need to get your blood pressure and pulse (heart rate) checked regularly.

Rimonabant (Acomplia)

Recently launched in the UK, rimonobant reduces appetite by blocking a chemical pathway in the brain known as the endocannabinoid system.

The endocannabinoid receptors were discovered by scientists looking for the binding sites for cannabis. Their role in appetite regulation was revealed when scientists noted that cannabis smokers developed food cravings and increased appetite, so they postulated that if the cannabis receptors were blocked then appetite might be reduced. The endocannabinoid system is also found in fat cells around our internal organs, and by blocking this system rimonabant may also reduce insulin resistance. Clinical trials have shown that rimonabant can enhance weight loss, reduce cholesterol, and improve insulin sensitivity. In the studies about 60 per cent of people taking rimonabant lost approximately 5 per cent of their initial body weight and about 30 per cent lost 10 per cent. People taking rimonabant lost on average 6 kg (13 lb) more than those on diet and exercise alone. Its main side effects are nausea, dizziness, diarrhoea, anxiety, and depression. You must not take it if you are thinking of becoming pregnant, are on antidepressants, or have a history of a mental illness.

Despite promising results, these drugs are still not the magic bullet that everyone is looking for. Not all patients respond to drug therapy and, as you can see, the medications can have side effects. Furthermore, once the drugs are stopped, most people tend to regain the weight they lost. The best way to lose weight is through long-term changes in your diet and by increasing your physical activity. Medication just makes these lifestyle changes more manageable for some.

Weight loss surgery

If you have a BMI of over 40, or over 35 and you have an obesity-related complication, and if you have tried lifestyle measures and prescription medication with little success, then surgery may be the final option. Surgery works by helping to reduce the number of calories that are available to your body either by reducing the size of the stomach so only small meals can be eaten and you feel full and/or by bypassing part of the small intestine so fewer calories from food are absorbed by the body. There are various operations available with different associated risks and benefits. The two most commonly performed operations are gastric banding and gastric bypass. Gastric banding involves putting a silicone tube around the upper half of the stomach, reducing the size of the stomach. A few weeks after the operation, the stomach size can be reduced further by injecting a small amount of fluid into the gastric band through the skin. Gastric bypass is a procedure whereby a small stomach pouch is formed at the top end of the stomach from which food is diverted away from the rest of the stomach through a newly formed exit into the end of the small intestine. Weight loss therefore occurs as a result of reduced food intake as the stomach size has been made smaller, and through reduced absorption as most of the small intestine is bypassed. Both operations are usually performed laparoscopically (keyhole surgery).

How much weight you lose will depend on both the type of operation you have and also on your willingness to change your eating and lifestyle habits after surgery. If you meet the medical criteria for weight loss surgery, the specialist unit will carefully assess your physical and emotional health before the decision to operate can be made. Weight loss surgery can be life changing for some people. Trials have shown that obesity surgery performed on the right person can result in the loss of 50–75 per cent excess body weight by 2 years after surgery and marked improvement or even resolution of diabetes and high blood pressure. Trials have also shown that weight loss following obesity surgery can result in a marked improvement in the symptoms of PCOS. However, it is not to be undertaken lightly—there is a risk of death of up to 1 per cent associated with the procedure as well as a risk of other complications.

We must stress that the operation will only help you eat less, and there is a lot required from you in reducing your food and calorie intake and increasing your physical activity after surgery if you want to lose weight. There is an excellent patient-led website which provides comprehensive information on the different types of weight loss surgery which we would recommend you look at if you have been referred for surgery or are considering your options (www.bospa.org.uk).

23

Weight maintenance—the bit 'diets' don't tell you

Key points

- Keeping weight off requires a different set of skills to losing weight.
- People who successfully lose weight and keep it off have certain characteristics, including eating breakfast, keeping active, and monitoring their weight and food intake.
- It is those people who take full responsibility for managing their own weight who are most successful in the long term.

Any diet that results in you eating fewer calories than you are burning off will result in weight loss. There are literally thousands of different diets on the bookshelves, each one with a different set of rules, which simply limit your choice of food so that you eat fewer calories. Most people, therefore, have managed to lose weight at some point in their lives. What these diet books do not teach you is how to keep the weight off once you have lost it. Keeping your weight the same (i.e. preventing future weight gain) requires a completely different set of skills from those needed when losing weight.

For one thing, when you are losing weight, you receive an abundance of positive feedback for your efforts. The scales show you that you are losing weight so you feel pleased with yourself. Your clothes begin to feel loose so you try on clothes that you haven't been able to fit into for years. This makes you feel fantastic and you deserve it. Your friends, especially those you haven't seen for a while, remark on how well you look and how great it is that you have lost so much weight.

When you are in the process of maintaining your weight, however, none of this positive feedback applies. No one says 'Wow your weight has so stayed the same—you look great, congratulations!' For this reason, the weight maintenance stage can be a frustrating time, as a lot of effort may still be required but for much smaller rewards.

What will help me keep off the weight I have lost?

As we discussed at the beginning of Part 3, diets don't work because people have unrealistic expectations of what they can achieve in terms of weight loss. This results in the development of overly restrictive eating behaviours to try to achieve the unrealistic rate of weight loss that people expect. This inevitably results in overcompensation, such as prolonged grazing or bingeing, whenever a lapse occurs. If you have a good understanding of the physics of weight loss from Chapter 15 of this book, then you should feel very proud of yourself whenever you have lost any weight at all, rather than feeling disappointed when you 'haven't lost enough'.

Most people lose weight for 12–15 weeks. If you have lost 5 per cent of your starting body weight in 12–15 weeks then you have been successful in the first stage. The hardest bit is keeping it off. As you know from Chapter 15, the heavier you are the more calories you burn off, so when you have lost weight you will burn off fewer calories than you did before you had lost that weight. If a 26-year-old inactive woman weighed 100 kg (15 stone 12 lb), she would burn off around 600 calories more than she would if she weighed 69 kg. This means that her energy expenditure would be reduced by 600 calories per day if she lost 5 stone.

Remember that, leading up to her weight loss, this woman must have been eating more calories than she was burning off to have enabled her to gain weight in the first place. In order for her to maintain her new lower weight, she would have to be prepared to eat at least 600 calories less than she was used to eating before she lost weight. This is an important point to remember, especially if you are someone that tends to 'go on a diet' and then go back to your old habits.

Clearly it would be much easier for someone gradually to get used to eating fewer calories rather than suddenly needing to eat considerably fewer calories. That is why we suggest that you try to lose weight in a stepwise fashion.

> Aim to lose 5 per cent of your body weight in 12–15 weeks and then adapt to your new lower weight for at least a month before attempting to lose your next 5 per cent.

This means that you need actively to try to stop losing weight and, instead, aim to keep your weight within 1 kg (2 lb) either side of the weight that you had achieved at the end of 12–15 weeks of weight loss. This will be very difficult for some of you, as you may still have a long way to go to reach your long-term weight loss goal. However, think about which will make you feel better in the long-term. Losing 3 stone in 6 months and then regaining 4 stone in the 6 months that follow? Or losing 3 stone in 1 year and still being 3 stone lighter in a year's time?

> It feels weird stopping trying to lose weight. I'm still 3 stone overweight and I've been trying to lose weight for as long as I can remember.

A study is being conducted in the USA, which people are asked to join if they have managed to lose 30 lb or more and have kept it off for a year. Around 4800 people have put their details on this National Weight Control Registry. These people have lost an average of 5 stone each and this has been maintained for an average of five and a half years—these people have been exceptionally successful at weight management. The investigators have asked each person about their lifestyles to discover what factors have helped them to keep the weight off that they have lost.

It emerged that they had all found different methods helpful in bringing about weight loss (including calorie-controlled diets, meal replacement programmes, and obesity surgery), but that they all had similar characteristics that caused them to keep the weight off once they had lost it.

The most common characteristics of people who have managed to maintain their weight loss are as follows.

1. They continue to eat breakfast almost every day.
2. They continue to eat a diet that is relatively low in fat.
3. They continue to monitor their food intake and body weight regularly by keeping a food diary periodically and weighing themselves once a week.
4. They continue to be physically active for approximately 60 minutes per day—for most people the chosen activity was walking.
5. Their daily calorie intake is fairly consistent throughout the week, i.e. they are not more restrictive on weekdays to allow themselves to have a blow-out each weekend.
6. Most people had previously made several unsuccessful attempts at maintaining their weight loss.

Breakfast

Certainly eating regularly was the most important factor shown to help people keep off the weight that they had lost. Interestingly, many of the women who come to our clinic say they struggle to eat breakfast. There seem to be some common reasons for this, including:

> I'm just not hungry in the mornings.
>
> I usually feel sick in the mornings.
>
> I can go all day without eating—but once I start I can't stop. So I'm worried that breakfast will set me up for eating constantly all day.
>
> I know I shouldn't skip breakfast but secretly I'm pleased with myself for skipping those calories.

It is worth bearing in mind the following facts.

- People who don't eat breakfast are much more likely to be overweight.
- People who skip breakfast feel more inclined to help themselves to biscuits when they pass the biscuit tin mid-morning because they feel they have 'saved' themselves calories by skipping breakfast. However, a bowl of breakfast cereal would have provided about 180 calories—they may have consumed this much after having only two biscuits from the tin.
- People who don't eat breakfast eat significantly more calories later in the day, particularly in the evenings.
- Because they eat more in the evenings, people who skip breakfast wake up in the morning still feeling full from the night before. It's no surprise then that they 'just don't feel like breakfast'.
- People who purposely try to avoid eating for as long as possible are setting themselves up to take in more calories in the long term. By going without food for a long period of time, you will develop an intense hunger. When we feel too hungry, we lose all control over what we are eating. For example, it is very common for women to get home from work feeling very hungry. They might start to prepare the dinner, but they often report eating half of the contents of the fridge whilst the dinner is cooking. When the dinner is finally ready, they have already eaten the caloric equivalent of a second dinner, so are not feeling very hungry anymore. However, on the principle that they have prepared the dinner, they eat it anyway. The problem in this case is that going too long without eating causes people to lose control when they do eat. This is easily rectified by planning snacks strategically during the day to prevent hunger.

My worst time of day is when I get home from work. How can I stop myself raiding the fridge?

Eating a relatively low-fat diet

Have you ever tried to follow a very strict low-fat diet and avoid all fatty foods? What usually happens is that people who restrict themselves too much end up eating much more of that food whenever they have a small lapse. See the section about 'dichotomous thinking' in Chapter 20 for more information about this.

The point is, if you tell yourself you're not allowed to eat any chocolate, you would be inclined to eat five bars at once rather than eat one bar. You would feel so guilty about eating one bar that you feel you have to 'get rid of the rest' to start again tomorrow! So by trying too hard to eat a low-fat diet, you may actually be eating a higher-fat diet. If you believe that you can eat any food you choose, then it's likely that you will naturally end up choosing a lower-fat diet, without really trying, because you won't be feeling guilty about eating anything.

People who are successful at maintaining their weight loss have learnt to think in a flexible way about food rather than in an 'all-or-nothing' way. People who consider themselves to be 'on a diet' and who consider certain foods to be 'naughty', will find it difficult to cope when the time comes that they do eat one of those foods.

Self-monitoring

As explained in detail in Chapter 17, those people who monitor their weight and food intake are more successful at maintaining weight loss. They weigh themselves once a week to keep an eye on their weight and, if they see that their weight is increasing, they keep a record of their food intake and activity, to try to find out what is causing the weight gain. To put it simply, it is those people who take full responsibility for their own weight who are most successful at controlling it in the long term.

Keeping active

As explained in Chapter 16, physical activity plays a very important role in weight maintenance. When you have lost weight, and in particular when you have lost lean tissue, the number of calories you burn each day will be slightly reduced. By keeping as active as possible, you can help to minimize this loss of lean tissue and therefore you can help your metabolic rate to decrease to a lesser extent. Some studies have demonstrated that people who incorporate physical activity into their daily lives (e.g. by walking to work or taking the stairs instead of the lift) maintain this increased level of activity for longer than those who take up structured activities such as aerobics classes or going to the gym.

Lapse management

Your ability to cope when you stray from your diet plan or when you don't manage to achieve your goals is likely to make the difference between managing your weight in the long term or starting the yo-yo dieting process all over again. This is why people who have successfully lost weight and kept it off tend to eat a consistent number of calories every day—they have learnt the skills needed to stop thinking in an all-or-nothing way. If they do go out for a meal at the weekend, they think of it as an opportunity to enjoy their favourite foods or to try some new foods, rather than thinking of it as an event which will ruin their 'diet'.

Don't give up

Many of the people who were successful enough at managing their weight to make it onto the National Weight Control Registry had a long history of numerous failed attempts at maintaining weight loss. Just because you have not been successful before does not mean that you should not be successful this time. You **can** do it!

Glossary

Acne: a skin condition characterized by greasy skin and spots on the face, neck, chest, and/or back caused by overproduction of oil by the sebaceous glands in the skin.

Adrenal glands: a pair of glands which lie just above each kidney and produce hormones such as cortisol which are essential for coping with stress and maintaining blood pressure. The adrenal glands also produce a small amount of androgens which are responsible for the development of pubic hair during puberty.

Alopecia: hair loss.

Amenorrhoea: failure to have a menstrual period for 6 months or more.

Androgens: sex hormones such as testosterone which are produced in abundance in males and result in male sexual characteristics. Small amounts are also produced in women and are essential for general well-being.

Anovulation: failure to ovulate, or release an egg every month for fertilization.

Anti-androgen: medication whch can be given to block the effects of androgens on the body.

Body mass index (BMI): a measurement of weight in kilograms divided by height in metres squared. A normal BMI is between 19 and 25 kg/m^2. A BMI below 19 kg/m^2 indicates that the person is underweight and a BMI above 25 kg/m^2 indicates that someone is overweight.

Cholesterol: a fatty substance made by the liver from saturated fats in food which plays an important role in cell function. However, too much cholesterol increases the risk of heart disease and stroke.

Combined contraceptive pill: contraceptive medication containing oestrogens and progestogens taken for three weeks out of every four. The high levels of oestrogens prevent ovulation and thus provide contraception, while the progestogen results in a withdrawal menstrual bleed every month. In addition to contraception, the combined pill may be used to regulate periods and to reduce period pains. Some pills, such as Dianette and Yasmin, may also reduce the effects of androgens on the skin.

Corpus luteum: the remainder of the ovarian follicle following release of the egg during ovulation. It is responsible for producing progesterone, a hormone which prepares the womb for implantation of the fertilized egg.

Cortisol: a hormone produced by the adrenal gland which is essential for life and for dealing with stress. It is one of the hormones which controls our blood pressure and energy levels. High levels of cortisol are produced during stressful events including severe illness. However, sustained high levels of cortisol are detrimental to health.

Dermatologist: a doctor who specializes in the treatment of skin disorders.

Diabetes: a condition resulting in high blood sugar levels. It is caused by the body not being able to produce enough insulin and/or not being able to use the insulin it produces efficiently.

Disaccharide: a type of carbohydrate made up of two sugar molecules bonded together, e.g. sucrose, lactose, and maltose.

Endocrine: the system in the body involved in the production and regulation of hormones.

Endocrinologist: a doctor who specializes in the treatment of endocrine disorders.

Endometrial hyperplasia: excessive growth of the lining of the womb due to exposure of the womb lining to oestrogen with lack of progesterone to counterbalance the oestrogen effects on endometrial growth. In women with PCOS this is usually caused by long-standing failure of ovulation which results in no progesterone production.

Endometrium: womb lining.

Follicle: egg-containing fluid-filled sacs produced in the ovaries. Usually, one follicle will mature every month, releasing an egg during ovulation.

Follicle-stimulating hormone (FSH): a hormone produced by the pituitary gland which controls ovarian follicle development and maturation and ovarian oestrogen production.

Gestational diabetes: diabetes that develops during pregnancy which tends to subside following childbirth. Women who develop gestational diabetes have an increased risk of developing type 2 diabetes.

Glucose: sugar produced from the breakdown of carbohydrates eaten which acts as a source of energy.

Glucose intolerance: abnormal blood sugar levels in response to a glucose load but not high enough to make the diagnosis of diabetes. Its presence indicates an increased risk of developing diabetes.

Glucose tolerance test: a test performed to diagnose diabetes and glucose intolerance. Fasting blood glucose level is taken, then the patient is given 75 g of a sugary substance to eat or drink, and blood sugar is measured 2 hours later.

Glycaemic index: a numerical calculation for carbohydrates based on their immediate effect on blood sugar levels. In general, the faster carbohydrates are digested, the higher the blood glucose response and the higher the glycaemic index.

Gynaecologist: a doctor who specializes in the treatment of infertility and the surgical treatment of disorders of the female reproductive organs.

HDL-cholesterol: a protein which removes cholesterol from the bloodstream. It is thought to protect against heart disease and stroke.

Hirsutism: excessive facial or body hair growth in a woman in a 'male-pattern' distribution. It is caused by higher than usual blood androgen levels or an increased sensitivity to androgens.

Hypertension: high blood pressure. If uncontrolled and untreated it can increase the risk of heart disease, stroke, and kidney disease.

Hyper-androgenism: a term indicating a higher than usual level of androgens in women

Hypothalamus: a tiny gland in the brain which lies just above the pituitary gland. It releases hormones which control the function of the pituitary gland and also plays a role in controlling appetite, body temperature, and sleep.

Hypothyroidism: underactivity of the thyroid gland, resulting in a slowing of metabolism and an increased propensity to weight gain.

Infertility: failure of a couple to conceive after trying for a year.

Insulin: a hormone produced by the pancreas which controls blood sugar levels by allowing the liver and muscle cells to take up glucose and use it as energy.

Insulin resistance: failure of the body to use insulin efficiently. As a result, excess amounts of insulin are produced in order to keep blood glucose levels within the normal range.

Insulin sensitizers: drugs such as metformin which act by making the cells of the body more responsive to insulin. Used to treat type 2 diabetes and more recently to treat some women with PCOS and insulin resistance.

Laparoscopy: an operation performed under a general anaesthetic whereby a telescope is inserted through a small incision just below the belly button and is used to inspect the ovaries, Fallopian tubes, and uterus. It is performed in women with infertility or pelvic pain to exclude blocked tubes, adhesions, or endometriosis.

LDL-cholesterol: a protein which transports cholesterol from the liver into the bloodstream. High levels are associated with narrowing of the arteries as a result of deposition of cholesterol in the arterial wall. This results in an increased risk of heart disease and stroke.

Luteinizing hormone (LH): a hormone produced by the pituitary gland which controls ovulation and stimulates androgen production by the ovaries.

Menses: periods.

Menstrual cycle: the hormonal changes that usually occur every month in women of childbearing age resulting in ovulation and preparation of the uterus for pregnancy. If pregnancy does not occur then the lining of the womb is shed at the end of the month, resulting in a period.

Metabolic syndrome: a term describing a group of abnormalities associated with insulin resistance. It is defined in the presence of abdominal fat deposition (a waist circumference of more than 80 cm in women) in addition to the presence of at least two of the following: high blood pressure, diabetes or abnormal glucose tolerance, and abnormal blood fats (low HDL-cholesterol and high tryglycerides). Its presence indicates an increased risk of developing diabetes and heart disease.

Monosaccharide: the name given to a carbohydrate made up of a single sugar molecule, e.g. glucose, fructose, and galactose

Obesity: accumulation of excess fat in the body resulting in a body weight which is 25 per cent above what is considered normal for your height. A BMI above 30 kg/m^2 is the measure most commonly used to diagnose obesity.

Oestrogen: a sex hormone normally produced in abundance in women, primarily by the ovaries, and responsible for the development of female sex characteristics. Small amounts are also normally produced in men.

Oligomenorrhoea: irregular menstrual periods occurring more than 40 days apart.

Osteoporosis: thinning of bones resulting in an increased risk of fractures, particularly in the spine and hips. More common in women after the menopause. Lack of oestrogens, smoking, and being underweight can increase the risk of developing osteoporosis in younger women.

Ovaries: two small glands lying in the pelvis close to the uterus which produce the sex hormones oestrogen, progesterone, and androgens. They also store and develop eggs.

Ovulation: the release of a matured egg from the follicle during the middle of the menstrual cycle in preparation for fertilization.

Pituitary gland: a small gland in the brain which releases hormones that regulate the function of the majority of the other endocrine glands in the body.

Progesterone: a sex hormone produced by the corpus luteum following ovulation. It prevents the release of more eggs and prepares the endometrial lining for implantation of a fertilized egg and pregnancy.

Progestogens: medications which have similar actions to progesterone.

Puberty: a term used to describe the physical and psychological changes that occur during sexual maturation from childhood to adulthood.

Sex hormone-binding globulin (SHBG): a protein produced by the liver and released into the bloodstream. The majority of sex hormones bind to SHBG and it is only the free hormones which are biologically active. Insulin resistance results in a suppression of SHBG production by the liver, with a resultant increase in circulating biologically active sex hormones. In contrast, the combined oral contraceptive pill increases SHBG production, thereby reducing the amount of free sex hormones.

Sebaceous glands: oil-producing glands connected to each hair follicle. Sebum, or oil, is produced and secreted through the skin pores to keep the skin and hair in good condition. However, too much sebum can result in blocked pores and acne.

Testosterone: the main male-type sex hormone produced by both men and women.

Triglycerides: a blood fat which is produced by fats in the diet. Too much triglyceride in the bloodstream can increase the risk of heart disease.

Uterus: the womb. A reproductive organ which carries a baby during pregnancy.

Appendix 1

Food and activity diary

When	Where and how	What and how much	Activity	Feelings
Sunday				
08:30	Standing up at the fridge	7 forkfuls of last night's left over Indian take-away		Starving—felt much better after eating that
08:45	Sitting at the kitchen table	1 large bowl of Coco Pops		Could've done without that as already felt satisfied by the curry
09:30			Went for a 30 min brisk walk with the dog	Felt guilty after too much breakfast—walk made me feel much better
10:00–12:30	Whilst doing housework	2 cups of tea (semi-skimmed milk, no sugar)		
13:00	Sitting at the kitchen table	1 sandwich—2 slices granary bread, low fat spread, 1/2 tin tuna, 1 tsp mayo, handful of salad, onions, peppers		Really enjoyed this. Feeling good about myself

Appendix 2

Progress chart

Date	Week no.	Weight	Waist	Hip	Change in weight, waist, or hip	How do I feel about myself?
	1					
	2					
	3					
	4					
	5					
	6					
	7					
	8					
	9					
	10					
	11					
	12					

Appendix 3

Calories used up during various activities

Activity	Intensity	Number of calories (kcal) burned per 30 min of activity at different body weight (kg)				
		60	**80**	**100**	**120**	**140**
Cleaning and dusting	Light	75	100	125	150	175
Painting/decorating	Moderate	90	120	150	180	210
Hoovering	Moderate	105	140	175	210	245
Golf	Moderate	129	180	225	270	315
Badminton	Moderate	174	234	291	350	404
Brisk walking, 4 mph	Moderate	150	234	285	337	389
Mowing the lawn	Moderate	165	220	275	330	385
Cycling, 5.5 mph	Moderate	115	150	190	230	265
Aerobic dancing	Moderate	135	180	225	270	315
Swimming slow crawl	Vigorous	240	320	400	480	560
Tennis, singles	Vigorous	240	327	400	480	560
Skipping rope	Vigorous	300	400	500	600	700
Running	Vigorous					
11 min/mile		240	327	400	480	560
8 min/mile		375	495	600	700	790

Data derived from: Ainsworth BE ***et al.*** (2000) Compendium of physical activities: an update of activity codes and MET intensities. *Medicine and Science in Sports and Exercise* 2000; 32(9 Suppl): S498–S504.

Appendix 4

What's a portion?

Fruit and vegetables	**1 unit (average 40 kcal)**
Dried fruit	1 matchbox size box raisins or 3 apricots, prunes, etc.
Fresh fruit, medium	1 whole fruit, e.g. 1 apple, 1 banana, 1 orange, 1 peach
Fresh fruit, large	1/2 a grapefruit or 1 slice of melon/pineapple
Fresh fruit, small	A large handful, e.g. 12 grapes, 2 medium plums, 2 kiwis, 7 strawberries, 3 clementines
Fruit juice (have no more than once daily)	1 small glass (125 ml) or small carton
Tinned fruit (in natural juice)	3 large tablespoons
Stewed fruit (no added sugar)	4 large tablespoons
Salad—mixed, e.g. lettuce, rocket, cucumber, peppers	1 small bowl
Tomato	1 large tomato or 10 cherry tomatoes
Vegetables, cooked, e.g. broccoli, cabbage, carrots, mushrooms, peas, peppers, tinned tomatoes	2 large tablespoons
Bread, other cereals and potatoes	**1 unit (approx 80 kcal)**
Breads and bread products	
Bagel	1/2 bagel
Bread or toast	1 medium slice (large loaf)
Bread roll	1/2 large roll

Chappati (made without fat)	1 small chapatti
Crackers, plain, e.g. cream crackers	3 crackers
Crispbreads, e.g. crackerbreads, rice cakes, Ryvita	4 crispbreads
Crumpet	1
English muffin	1/2 muffin
Naan bread, plain	1/2 naan bread = 3 units
Pitta bread	1 mini or 1/2 large pitta
Breakfast cereals	
Flakes or crispies	3 tablespoons
Muesli	2 tablespoons
Muesli bar	1 bar
Porridge oats (dry)	3 tablespoons
Shredded Wheat or Weetabix	1
Noodles, rice, and pasta	
Egg noodles, boiled	1/2 serving
Pasta, plain (white or wholemeal), boiled	3 heaped tablespoons
Plantain (green banana)	1/2 small plantain
Potatoes (no added fat)	2 egg-size potatoes or 1/2 medium baked potato
Rice, plain (white or wholemeal)	2 heaped tablespoons
Yam (boiled)	1/2 medium yam
Milk and dairy products	**1 unit (average 90 kcal)**
Cheeses	
Cottage cheese	1/2 a 227 g carton
Cheddar and hard cheeses*	1/2 matchbox-size piece (20 g)
Cream cheese—full fat*	1/8 of a 225 g tub
–light*	1/4 of a 200 g tub
–extra light	1/3 of a 200 g tub
Lower fat cheeses*, e.g. Brie, Camembert, Edam, Feta, Mozzarella, reduced fat Cheddar	1 matchbox-size piece (30 g)

Creams	
Crème fraiche, full-fat*	1 tablespoon
Crème fraiche, half-fat*2 large tablespoons	
Double cream*	1 tablespoon
Single cream*	3 level tablespoons
Fromage frais, low fat	1 small pot (100 g)
Milks	
Semi-skimmed (or unsweetened soya milk)	1 medium glass (200 ml)
Skimmed	1 large glass (250 ml)
Whole	1 small glass (135 ml)
Yoghurts	
Greek-style yoghurt, full fat*	1/2 small (150 g) pot
Plain or flavoured, low calorie/diet	1 large individual pot (200 g)
Plain or flavoured, low fat	2/3 of a small (150 g) pot
Meat, fish and alternatives	**1 unit (approx 150 kcal)**
Eggs	2
Fish	
Fish fingers	3
Oily fish, e.g. mackerel, salmon, sardines, trout, tuna (fresh)	1 medium fillet or steak (100 g)
Oily fish, tinned in tomato sauce	3/4 of a 125 g tin
Seafood—prawns, mussels, scallops	1/2 a 300 g packet
Seafood (crab flavour) sticks	10 sticks
White fish (e.g. cod, haddock) or tinned tuna in brine	1 large fillet or steak (150 g)
Meat	
Lean meat, e.g. beef, ham, lamb, lean mince, pork (with fat removed)	3 small slices (75 g)
Lean poultry—chicken, turkey (without skin)	A piece the size of a pack of playing cards (85 g)
Nuts	1/2 a small packet (25 g)

Peanut butter	1 tablespoon (25 g)
Pulses	
Baked beans in tomato sauce (reduced sugar and salt)	1/2 a 400 g tin
Pulses, cooked, e.g. chick peas, butter beans, kidney beans, lentils	4 tablespoons
Houmous	1/6 of a 300 g pot
Quorn or soya products, e.g. mince, burger, sausage	1 serving or about 100 g
Fatty and sugary foods	**1 unit (average 60 kcal)**
Butter* or margarine	1 teaspoon
Low-fat spread (40 % fat)	2 teaspoons
Mayonnaise	1 teaspoon
Mayonnaise, reduced calorie	2 teaspoons
Oil (any type)	2 level teaspoons
Salad cream	1 tablespoon
Salad cream, reduced calorie	2 tablespoons

Extras worth about 50 kcal
◆ One extra piece of fruit (except bananas)
◆ Crunchy vegetables with salsa dip
◆ 1 small (125 g) pot of low-calorie yoghurt
◆ 1 crispbread or rice cake with 1 slice of wafer thin ham and tomato
◆ 2 Tuc or water biscuits
◆ 1 Jaffa Cake, gingernut, rich tea, Garibaldi biscuit or fig-roll
◆ 1 cup of low-calorie hot chocolate drink
◆ 1 Slim-A-Soup
◆ 1 fancy chocolate*
◆ 2 1/2 teaspoons of sugar 1 packet of sugar-free Polo mints 1 mini-milk lolly

Extras worth about 100 kcal
• 1 banana
• Crunchy vegetables with 1/4 pot of guacamole or tzatziki dip
• 1 slice of bread or toast (medium thick) with thinly spread jam or marmalade (use fat spread from allowance)
• 1 medium-sized (200 g) pot of low-calorie yoghurt, e.g. Mullerlite
• 1 small packet of corn snacks e.g. Skips*, Wotsits*, Quavers*
• 1 packet of Twiglets
• 3 tablespoons of breakfast cereal
• 1 Kitkat*
• 1 cereal bar
• 1 plain or chocolate digestive* or Hobnob*
• 1 shortbread finger*
• 1 fun-size chocolate bar
• 2 fancy chocolates*
• 1 glass of semi-skimmed milk
• 1/2 pint of lager
• 1 medium glass of wine
Extras worth about 150 kcal
• 1 slice of bread or toast (medium thick) with ordinary butter* or margarine
• 1 slice of toast (without fat spread) with 'light' soft cheese*
• 1 picnic size pitta bread with 25 g houmous
• 1 currant bun
• 1 oatcake with full-fat cream cheese* or thickly spread 'light' cream cheese*
• 1 packet of reduced-fat potato crisps*
• 1/4 of a 100 g packet of peanuts

- 1/6 of a tube of Pringles*
- 1 cup of hot chocolate (made with 200 ml semi-skimmed milk and 3 tsp drinking chocolate powder)
- 1 Penguin bar*
- 1/2 of a large American-style cookie*
- 1 cereal bar
- 3 fancy chocolates*
- 1 choc ice or Solero ice cream

Extras worth about 200 kcal

- Crunchy vegetables with 1/6 of a small pot of houmous or sour-cream dip
- 1 bowl of cereal (30 g) with semi-skimmed milk
- 1 slice of toast (without fat spread) with 20 g of hazelnut chocolate spread
- 1 slice of toast (without fat spread) with 20 g of peanut butter
- 1 slice of toast (without fat spread) with 40 g of 'light' soft cheese
- 1 cream cracker with 1 matchbox-sized (40 g) piece of cheese*
- 1 packet (30g) of ordinary potato crisps*
- 1 small slice of fruit cake or sponge
- 1 plain or fruit scone (use spread from allowance)
- 1 ordinary packet of Maltesers*, M&Ms* or Smarties*
- 1 Crunchie bar or 'flake'-type chocolate bar*
- 2 fun-size chocolate bars
- 4 fancy chocolates*
- 10 jelly babies

*Foods marked with an asterisk contain a large amount of saturated fat or sugar. You should be able to enjoy these foods in moderation but take care with the amounts.

Appendix 5

Calorie content of alcoholic drinks

	Calorie content	Units of alcohol
Champagne—115 ml flute	80 kcal	1
Dry white wine		
◆ 125 ml glass	81 kcal	1
◆ 175 ml glass	114 kcal	1.5
◆ 250 ml glass	163 kcal	2
Medium white wine		
◆ 125 ml glass	98 kcal	1
◆ 175 ml glass	137 kcal	1.5
◆ 250 ml glass	195 kcal	2
Red wine		
◆ 125 ml glass	88 kcal	1
◆ 175 ml glass	123 kcal	1.5
◆ 250 ml glass	175 kcal	2
Ordinary strength lager, e.g. Carling, Fosters		
◆ 1/2 pint	91 kcal	1
◆ 1 pint	182 kcal	2
◆ 440 ml can	176 kcal	1.5

	Calorie content	Units of alcohol
Premium lager, e.g. Stella, Kronenbourg		
◆ 1/2 pint	120 kcal	1.5
◆ 1 pint	239 kcal	3
◆ 440 ml can	185 kcal	2.3
◆ 275 ml bottle	116 kcal	1.5
Strong lager—440 ml can	330 kcal	4
Bitter		
◆ 1/2 pint	102 kcal	1
◆ 1 pint	204 kcal	2
◆ 440 ml can	158 kcal	1.5
Sweet cider		
◆ 1/2 pint	180 kcal	1
◆ 1 pint	360 kcal	2
Dry cider		
◆ 1/2 pint	100 kcal	1
◆ 1 pint	200 kcal	2
◆ 440 ml can	156 kcal	1.5
Alcopop—250 ml bottle	250 kcal	1.5
Fortified wines—50 ml measures		
◆ Dry sherry	54 kcal	1
◆ Medium sherry	58 kcal	1
◆ Cream sherry	63 kcal	1
◆ White port	70 kcal	1
◆ Vintage port	80 kcal	1
Generic spirits—25 ml measures		
◆ Brandy	50 kcal	1
◆ Gin	50 kcal	1
◆ Rum	50 kcal	1
◆ Vodka	50 kcal	1
◆ Whisky	50 kcal	1

	Calorie content	Units of alcohol
Branded spirits		
◆ Bacardi—25 ml measure	50 kcal	1
◆ Jack Daniels—25 ml measure	60 kcal	1
◆ Pernod—25 ml measure	61 kcal	1
◆ Pimms—50 ml measure	98 kcal	1
◆ Southern Comfort—25 ml measure	70 kcal	1
Liqueurs		
◆ Baileys—50 ml measure	160 kcal	1
◆ Benedictine—25 ml measure	90 kcal	1
◆ Cointreau—25 ml measure	85 kcal	1
◆ Drambuie—25 ml measure	85 kcal	1
◆ Tia Maria—25 ml measure	75 kcal	1

Appendix 6

Relative glycaemic index of some common foods

Low GI Best choices	Medium GI OK choices	High GI Is there a lower GI alternative?
Beans and pulses, including baked beans		
White or wholemeal wheat pasta	Rice noodles	Rice pasta
Wheat noodles	Gnocchi	
Soya and linseed bread Rye bread Oat bread	Granary or multigrain bread Pitta bread—white or wholemeal Stoneground wholemeal sourdough bread Chapatti	White bread Wholemeal bread
Sweet potato, baked Yam, boiled	Tinned new potatoes	Instant mashed potato Mashed potato Jacket potato Boiled old or new potatoes
Pearl barley	White basmati rice Wild rice White long-grain rice	Jasmine rice White glutinous rice
All-Bran	Special K	Rice Krispies, Coco pops
Muesli		Cornflakes, Crunchy Nut Cornflakes

Low GI Best choices	Medium GI OK choices	High GI Is there a lower GI alternative?
Porridge		Branflakes, Sultana Bran Shredded Wheat
Oat cakes	Ryvita	Rice cakes Puffed crispbread Melba toast
Oatmeal biscuits Rich tea	Digestives Shortbread	Morning coffee
Low-calorie or diet drinks Milk—all types Fruit juices	Cola, original Fruit squash, original	Lucozade original
Artificial sweeteners, e.g. Splenda, Canderel, Sweetex, Hermesetes Fructose Honey	Sucrose Golden syrup	Glucose

With the exception of low-calorie or diet drinks, milk, and artificial sweeteners, the foods in the shaded area are either high in saturated fat or sugar, so are not necessarily 'healthy' or helpful to those who are trying to lose weight. They are simply given on this table so that comparisons can be made.

Appendix 7

List of useful websites

Polycystic ovary syndrome

www.verity-pcos.org.uk—The UK PCOS patient support group

www.pcos-uk.org.uk

www.pcosupport.org—The American PCOS Patient support group

www.soulcysters.com—an American patient-led site with an active forum

Weight and nutrition

www.bda.uk.com—British Dietetic Association

www.bdaweightwise.com

www.nutrition.org.uk—British Nutrition Foundation

www.nutritionsociety.org

www.eatwell.gov.uk—Food Standards Agency website for food and health

www.glycemicindex.com—comprehensive database on GI contents of foods

www.caloriesperhour.com—useful site for information on caloric content of food and calories burnt per physical activity

www.weightlossresources.co.uk—a subscription site to help guide weight loss

www.weightwatchers.co.uk

www.slimming-world.co.uk

www.nationalobesityforum.org.uk

www.bospa.org.uk—British Obesity Surgery Patients Association

www.wlsinfo.org.uk—patient-led site with active forum on obesity surgery

www.toast-uk.org—The Obesity Awareness and Solutions Trust

Herbal medicine

www.nimh.org.uk—National Institute of Medical Herbalists

Diabetes

www.diabetes.org

www.diabetes.org.uk

Heart disease

www.bhf.org—British Heart Foundation website

Fertility

www.fertilityfriends.co.uk—patient-led support group

www.zitawest.com

www.infertilitynetworkuk.com

Hirsutism

www.electrolysis.co.uk

www.healthcarecommission.org.uk

Hair loss

www.alopecia-awareness.org.uk

www.alopeciaonline.org.uk

Acne

www.stopspots.org

General patient information

www.patient.co.uk

www.netdoctor.co.uk

www.nhsdirect.nhs.uk

Index